METHODS IN IMMUNODIAGNOSIS

a volume in the series

TECHNIQUES IN
PURE AND APPLIED MICROBIOLOGY

edited by

CARL-GÖRAN HEDÉN

Karolinska Institute, Stockholm

METHODS IN IMMUNODIAGNOSIS

EDITED BY

NOEL R. ROSE

AND

PIERLUIGI E. BIGAZZI

Center for Immunology
State University of New York at Buffalo

A WILEY-INTERSCIENCE PUBLICATION

JOHN WILEY & SONS
New York • London • Sydney • Toronto

Library of Congress Cataloging in Publication Data:

Rose, Noel R.
     Methods in immunodiagnosis.
     (Techniques in pure and applied microbiology)
     "A Wiley-Interscience publication."

     1. Immunohemotology. 2. Serum diagnosis.
I. Bigazzi, Pierluigi E., joint author. II. Title.
III. Series. [DNLM: 1. Immunologic techniques.
QY 250 M592 1973]

RB45.R67   616.07'56   73–646

ISBN 0-471-73520-5

Printed in the United States of America

10 9 8 7 6 5 4 3 2 1

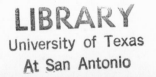

SERIES PREFACE

This series of handbooks is an effort to supply the practical advice that is needed in most laboratories active in the various fields of applied microbiology and to do it without an overdose of theoretical considerations. This, however, does not imply that the books will be of only limited value to a theoretically oriented laboratory. Consider the extensive use of microorganisms as research tools—now common among biophysicists, molecular biologists, immunologists, bioengineers and many others—and you will appreciate the need for a quick guide to the accepted techniques for handling bacteria and viruses.

Pure and applied microbiology go together; they are opposite sides of the same coin. The former is a road over forbiddingly steep hills on which the path is always partly hidden from view. The latter is the goal, for, after all, as Orville Wyss has emphasized, applied microbiology constitutes the backbone of our science, even if "we have responded to the gibes of the humanists who have always objected to the university leaving the cloister and entering the market place. It has never been demonstrated that the cloister is in any way superior to the market place for training a man to think, or that applied science is in any way inferior to pure science as an intellectual effort." There are many signs that the young student generation is more keenly aware of this than most of their professors, but this should not make the students forget Louis Pasteur's famous statement: "Without theory, practice is but routine born of habit. Theory alone can bring forth and develop the spirit of inventions." If the student keeps this in mind he will find that microbiology offers more challenging opportunities to make inventions that will affect man's future health and well-being than most other subjects which he might choose to study.

Carl-Göran Hedén

Introduction

The term "immunodiagnosis" has been selected to denote the many applications of immunological methods to the diagnosis of human disease. To our minds, it is more appropriate than the older term, "serodiagnosis," because some of the most important procedures use reactions of cell-mediated, rather than humoral, immunity. Moreover, the approach depends upon the immune response, not upon serum per se.

The immune response lends itself to diagnostic applications because of its two outstanding properties of sensitivity and specificity. Sensitivity refers to the ability of immunological reagents-antibodies or cellular receptors, or the secondary reactors such as complement or histamine-to respond to extremely small amounts of antigen. Often microgram or picogram amounts will suffice to initiate a detectable response.

The specificity of immunological reactions allows one to demonstrate with ease differences that are difficult to show by even the most precise methods of biochemical analysis. A single difference in an amino acid or monosaccharide unit may be recognized by properly selected antisera.

The earliest applications of immunological diagnosis centered around the demonstration of circulating antibodies to pathogenic microorganisms. The French physician Widal pointed out that one could arrive indirectly at a diagnosis of typhoid fever by showing specific agglutinins in the bloodstream. Even more convincing evidence comes from finding a rising titer in serum samples taken during convalescence as compared with the acute phase. This principle underlies most of classical serology. The methods are useful even if the causative agent is unavailable, provided an appropriate related antigenic determinant can be found. For instance, the Wassermann test depends upon a widely distributed cardiolipin; the Weil-Felix reaction upon an antigen shared by Rickettsia and proteins; and the cold hemagglutination test upon a heterogenetic reaction with a human erythrocyte antigen. The demonstration of antibodies is of special importance in the diagnosis of many viral infections and in the determination of safe transfusion. Antibodies to foreign antigens may point to hypersensitivity or allergic disorders where antibodies to autologous antigens can be used as markers for autoimmune diseases.

The use of antibodies for the recognition of bacterial antigens was first proposed by Gruber and Durham. They could easily differentiate typhoid from cholera organisms in specific agglutination reactions with defined antisera. Today, this basic concept is applied for the indentification of many pathogenic microorganisms and for the recognition of antigens of erythrocytes, leukocytes, and other tissue cells. Moreover, the immunological method lends itself to the precise quantitative analysis of many bodily constituents, including the immunoglobulins and other plasma proteins, circulating peptide or steroid hormones, or drugs.

Immunodiagnostic methods find special application in the study of disorders of the immunological system itself. Malignancy of lymphoreticular cells may result in an unbalanced production of immunoglobulin components; genetic defects may depress production of circulating antibodies, or the function of lymphocytes, macrophages, circulating phagocytes, or complement. Abnormal immunological reactivity may cause allergic or autoimmune disease.

Because of the rising importance of methods of immunodiagnosis, the Immunology Unit of the World Health Organization (WHO) encouraged its Regional Reference Center for autoimmune serology in Buffalo to offer a laboratory course in this field. In 1969, the Center for Immunology, parent organization of the Reference Center, prepared a three-week laboratory-oriented Summer School in Methods of Research in Immunodiagnosis. It attracted clinical laboratory physicians and scientists from North and South America, Europe, Asia, and Africa. The course was repeated in 1971.

The course drew upon the experience and skill of all members of the immunological community in Buffalo, which comprises the Center for Immunology. This volume is derived from the laboratory guide designed for the Summer School. It represents the combined efforts of the Buffalo group. In two specific areas, radioimmunoassay and complement measurement, assistance was sought from outside experts.

While assembling this book, the editors were keenly aware of the extraordinarily rapid growth of the field of immunodiagnosis. Even during the preparation process, some methods, such as the radioimmunoassay for carcinoembryonic antigen, became so widely adopted that they could justify a place in the volume. Obviously, it was necessary to make some arbitrary selections. We have attempted to emphasize those procedures that are not extensively described in existing books of immunochemical methods and to present the underlying principles that are broadly applicable to immunodiagnosis.

Buffalo, New York
December, 1972

Noel R. Rose
Pierluigi E. Bigazzi

Contributors

Dr. C. Abeyounis
Department of Microbiology
State University of New York
at Buffalo

Dr. G. Andres
Departments of Pathology
and Microbiology
State University of New York
at Buffalo

Dr. A. Barron
Department of Microbiology
State University of New York
at Buffalo
and Erie County Virology Laboratory

Dr. W. Bartholomew
Department of Microbiology
State University of New York
at Buffalo

Dr. P. Bigazzi
The Center for Immunology and
Department of Microbiology
State University of New York
at Buffalo

Dr. S. Cohen
Department of Pathology and
The Center for Immunology
State University of New York
at Buffalo

Dr. H. Fuji
Department of Microbiology
State University of New York
at Buffalo

Dr. E. Gorzynski
Department of Microbiology
State University of New York
at Buffalo
and Assistant Director of
the Public Health Division
of Erie County Laboratory

Mr. S. Gutcho
Associate Director of Research and
Development-Radioimmunoassay
Schwarz/Mann Company

Dr. K. Kano
Department of Microbiology
State University of New York
at Buffalo

Dr. J. Kite
Department of Microbiology
State University of New York
at Buffalo

Dr. R. Lambert
Department of Microbiology
State University of New York
at Buffalo

Dr. F. Milgrom
Department of Microbiology
State University of New York
at Buffalo

Dr. J. Mohn
Department of Microbiology
State University of New York
at Buffalo

Dr. J. Puleo
Department of Microbiology
State University of New York
at Buffalo
and Director of Public Health Division
of Erie County Laboratory

Dr. B. Rabin
Department of Pathology
University of Pittsburgh

Dr. N. Rose
The Center for Immunology and
Department of Microbiology
State University of New York
at Buffalo

Dr. C. J. van Oss
Department of Microbiology
State University of New York
at Buffalo

Dr. K. Wicher
Department of Microbiology
State University of New York
at Buffalo and
Director of Clinical Microbiology
of Erie County Laboratory

Dr. R. Zarco
Associate Director of
Biochemical Research
Cordis Laboratories

Dr. R. Zeschke
The Center for Immunology and
Department of Microbiology
State University of New York
at Buffalo

Contents

Chapter 1

PRECIPITATION REACTIONS

C. J. van Oss   B. Rabin
P. Bigazzi   W. Bartholomew
A. Barron   K. Wicher

When a soluble antigen and its antibody contact each other in solution, the resulting antigen-antibody complexes may become insoluble and precipitate. The precipitation rate depends on the proportions of the reactants and on the temperature, salt concentration, and, to some extent, the pH of the solution.

The precipitation reaction can be produced by mixing antigen and antibody in test tubes or in Lang-Levy pipettes. It can also be obtained by carefully overlaying one reactant with the other in a narrow test tube so that diffusion can take place; the antigen-antibody reaction is then visible as a precipitation ring at the liquid interface. The Swift-Wilson-Lancefield precipitation test can be considered a combination of the two previous techniques. It is performed in capillary tubes, and precipitation is initially observed at the interface but later also in the lower part of the tubes, since mixture by convection occurs.

A precipitation reaction can be performed by allowing antigen and antibody to diffuse in gels. When one reactant diffuses into a gel containing the other reactant, the reaction is defined as a single (or simple) diffusion. Single-diffusion methods are performed in tubes (Oudin technique) or, more commonly, in plates (radial immunodiffusion or the Mancini technique). When both antigen and antibody diffuse into a gel that initially did not contain either one, the reaction is defined as double diffusion. Double-diffusion methods are performed in tubes (one-dimension or single-dimension double diffusion, the Oakley and Fulthorpe or Preer technique) or more commonly in plates (two-dimension double diffusion, the Elek or Ouchterlony technique).

The use of electrophoresis prior to two-dimension double diffusion in agar was first introduced by Grabar and Williams, who designated it "immunoelectrophoretic analysis." Other variations have since been proposed, such as the use of electrophoresis both preliminary to and during single diffusion in agar (two-dimensional, "crossed" immunoelectrophoresis) or just during single diffusion

1

(electroimmunodiffusion). Another modification makes use of the endosmotic flow, which, during electrophoresis in a negatively charged gel, causes the slow-moving γ globulins to be displaced toward the cathode, that is, in a direction opposite to the fast-moving antigen. By appropriate arrangement of wells, antigen and antibody can be made to converge (immunoelectroosmophoresis or "crossover" electrophoresis). The efficiency of the double-diffusion precipitation reaction can also be improved, bringing antigen and antibody together by hydrodynamic transport through the continuous evaporation of water from the gel in the spot where the precipitation reaction is to take place (immunorheophoresis).

The sensitivity of the precipitation reactions in gels can be increased using special stains for proteins or, when feasible, stains for enzymes. Very weak reactions can also be detected by autoradiography of precipitation reactions in which either antigen or antibody had been labeled with radioisotopes.

The use of immunoprecipitation techniques in a diagnostic laboratory provides the capability of diagnosing and following the course of patients with various immunological and nonimmunological disorders. Examples of diagnosis by the simple observation of an antigen using two-dimensional diffusion are the detection of α-fetoprotein and of the hepatitis-associated antigen. Quantitative abnormalities in the serum concentration of proteins are exemplified by the lowering of haptoglobin in hemolytic anemia, of antitrypsin in chronic obstructive lung disease, and of immunoglobulins in immune-deficiency diseases. The quantitative abnormalities are assayed by using the technique of quantitative radial immunodiffusion.

Both qualitative and quantitative techniques become important in diagnosing plasma cell dyscrasias. The homogeneous serum protein is often first detected by serum protein electrophoresis, but the definitive identification and confirmation that it is homogeneous depends on immunoelectrophoresis. Quantitation of the homogeneous and noninvolved immunoglobulin classes by radial immunodiffusion is then used to follow the course of the patient and to add to the information needed to classify the patient in a benign or malignant category.

PRECIPITATION IN CAPILLARY TUBES

Precipitation reactions performed in capillary tubes have the advantage of requiring very small amounts of reagents in comparison to the reactions in regular test tubes. This test was introduced by Swift, Wilson and Lancefield to test for the presence of M substance in steptococci but has also been used to detect pneumococcal carbohydrates and C-reactive protein. It can be employed to detect soluble antigens generally and to titrate their antibodies.

Materials

1. Disposable capillary tubes (75 mm x 1.04-1.24 mm internal diameter)
2. Antiserum
3. Soluble antigen } Both reagents should be clear. Centrifuge if necessary.
4. Support with modeling clay (wooden block in which a groove is cut and filled with modeling clay; immunodiffusion plate filled with clay; glass slide covered with clay; holders for microhematocrit capillary tubes)

Method

1. Fill one-third of capillary tube with antiserum.
2. Wipe outside of tube with moist tissue paper.
3. Draw up an equal volume of antigen solution.
4. Wipe again the outside of the tube.
5. Admit a small amount of air into the tube. No air bubbles should get between antiserum and antigen.
6. Close top end of tube with forefinger, then stick tube into modeling clay contained in support. Precipitation will start within seconds, but a longer time is required for complete precipitation.
7. Let stand at room temperature for one hour; then read.
8. Leave tubes overnight in refrigerator and read again.
9. Reactions can be graded as just visible (±), a few fine masses visible with a lens (+), easily seen without a lens (++), or capillary filled with masses of precipitate (+++ to ++++). When a compact precipitate is obtained, the height of the column of precipitate in each tube can also be measured in millimeters (mm).
10. Sometimes it is desirable to test varying concentrations of antigen to avoid surplus inhibition.

REFERENCES

1. Anderson, H. C. and McCarty, M. Determination of C-reactive protein in the blood as a measure of the activity of the disease process in acute rheumatic fever. *Am. J. Med. 8*, 445 (1950).
2. Swift, H. F., Wilson, A. T., and Lancefield, R. C. Typing group A hemolytic streptococci by M precipitin reactions in capillary pipettes. *J. Exptl. Med. 78*, 127 (1943).

DOUBLE DIFFUSION IN TWO DIMENSIONS (OUCHTERLONY)

Double-diffusion methods make use of the fact that antigens and their antibodies, upon meeting after double diffusion in a gel, tend to form a precipitate band that is specifically impermeable to the antigen and antibody that formed it. The precipitate band (or as seen from above, the precipitate line) is permeable to all other antigens and antibodies that have no points of identity with the first pair.

Therefore, two identical antigens (or antibodies) diffusing from two different wells, when reacted with their antibody (or antigen) diffusing from a third well, will form precipitate lines at an angle with one another that will fuse (reaction of identity, Fig. 1.1.A). Under the same conditions two antigens that have nothing in common, when reacted with their antibodies, mixed together and diffusing from one well against them, will form two precipitate lines, at an angle with one another that will cross (reaction of nonidentity, Fig. 1.1.B). These two situations can also occur together, in cases of partial identity. Precipitate lines that partly cross and partly fuse are then seen, resulting in a pattern that has come to be called a spur (Figs. 1.1.C and D).

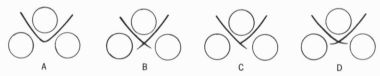

Fig. 1.1. Basic reaction patterns in double-diffusion methods (1 and 2: antigen wells; 3: antibody wells).

Quantitative antigen-antibody titrations can be performed with the gel-precipitation double-diffusion method owing to the fact that the precipitate band always first forms in the same place between the wells, depending only on the diffusion constants of the reagents and not on their concentrations. It will remain specifically impermeable to the antigen and antibody that formed it only as long as equivalent amounts of both reagents remain present in solution on either side of the band. When one of the reagents, say, the antigen, is much more concentrated than the antibody, it will be able to cross the precipitate line and diffuse further toward the antibody well, thus causing either a thickening of the precipitate line in the direction of the antibody, which was present in a lower concentration, or an apparent displacement of the entire precipitate line in that direction. Thus, titrations can be set up where a thin, sharp, unmoved line is indicative of the equivalence zone, while thickened lines or lines that have moved occur in all places of nonequivalence, the thickening or moving of the lines being in the direction of the reagent present in the lower concentration.

Double-diffusion techniques have been used for studies of bacterial and viral antigens and for the detection of antibodies to several microorganisms but are not routinely used in clinical microbiology. However, several laboratories that have developed the method for viral antigens have found it very useful for presumptive diagnosis. The procedure is not particularly sensitive but has been used to detect antibodies in a number of different viral infections. Antibodies to herpes simplex, varicella, enteroviruses, and influenza have been demonstrated by diffusion of patients' sera against the corresponding antigens. The method may also be used for the detection of viral antigens, as exemplified in cases of variola (smallpox), where large amounts of antigen accumulate in the lesions and can be easily examined. A major contribution of the procedure has been the detection of the hepatitis-associated antigen (HAA or Australia antigen) in the serum of patients with viral hepatitis and in blood donors. Even though at present counterimmunoelectrophoresis is routinely used for the demonstration of HAA (p. 19), the double-diffusion procedure is still employed to confirm the results obtained with counterimmunoelectrophoresis or other methods.

The Ouchterlony procedure is also used to detect the presence of α-feto-protein (fetoglobulin), a protein normally absent in adult human serum but present in the serum of many patients with liver tumors. The test is especially useful for screening patients with cirrhosis of the liver in which a hepatoma may be suspected. Positive reactions are also obtained in a certain percentage of patients with testicular tumors, but from a clinical diagnostic point of view these positive reactions do not actually interfere with the diagnosis of primary liver tumor. The reaction can in fact also be used to confirm the presence of a testicular tumor.

Many variations of the double-diffusion technique have been described, and they can be distinguished as macromethods and micromethods and according to the different kinds of containers for the gel (petri dishes, glass plates, microscope slides), different shapes and volumes of the wells and different kinds of gels (agar of various purity, pectin, sodium alginate).

One macromethod and one micromethod will be described. The latter is a modification that has the advantage of using approximately 0.02 milliliters (ml) of each reactant per test, while many macromethods require 5-10 times more.

Macro Double-Diffusion Test (Ouchterlony)

Materials

1.   Special agar, 1% (p. 207)
2.   Phosphate-buffered saline solution, pH 7.2, 1.5 M (PBS)

3.   Bovine serum albumin solution (BSA)
4.   Rabbit antiserum to BSA
5.   Amido black or Ponceau red stains (pp. 196, 206)
6.   Absorbent paper
7.   Acetic acid, 1 M
8.   Pasteur pipettes
9.   Plastic disposable petri dishes (50 x 12 mm or 100 x 15 mm)

Method

1.   Fill the petri dishes, on a level surface, with warm (50-60°C) special agar, using 3 ml for 50 x 12 mm dishes or 12 ml for 100 x 15 mm dishes.
2.   Swirl the dish gently until the agar is evenly spread over the bottom of the dish. Cover.
3.   Allow to set at least 20 minutes. Refrigerate until use.
4.   Upon use, punch out the desired pattern. (Wells are punched out of the agar using small cork borers, cut-off needles, or commercially available cutters. A wide variety of patterns of wells may be employed.)
5.   Remove agar from wells with suction.
6.   Fill wells with desired reagents using Pasteur pipettes. Cover the dish and allow the reagents to diffuse about 24 hours at room temperature, on a level surface.
7.   Read with the aid of oblique illumination. Results may be drawn or photographed against a dark background with side lighting.
8.   Stain the plates. a. Immerse petri dishes in a pan of saline solution for two to three days, with two or three daily changes of saline in order to remove the unprecipitated antigen and antiserum. b. After rinsing with water, a piece of wetted absorbent paper is placed in the dish so that no air is trapped between the agar surface and the paper. c. The dish is dried overnight in a 37°C incubator and the paper is peeled away from the film of agar. d. The precipitates are then stained with a protein stain such as Ponceau red or amido black for 10-20 minutes and decolorized in three baths of 1M acetic acid until the background turns clear. e. After rinsing once with water, the dishes are air dried and stored.

Micro Double-Diffusion Test (Wadsworth)

Materials

1.   Cleansed glass slides (50 x 50 mm or 50 x 75 mm) are coated with an agar film by spreading about 0.2-0.3 ml of 0.3% agar (prepared in distilled

water) over the slide. Coated slides are dried in an oven or incubator.

2. Antiserum
3. Antigen
4. Special agar, 1% (p. 207)
5. Templates are prepared from pieces of Plexiglass (38 x 40 x 3 mm) by drilling holes arranged in a suitable pattern. These holes are 3 mm in diameter but with an aperture at the lower surface of 2 mm. Strips of waterproof tape not more than 4 mm wide are applied to the lower surface on opposite sides of the matrix to provide a chamber of the desired depth (0.4-0.8 mm) (see Fig. 1.2.)
6. Pasteur pipettes and 1-ml pipettes
7. Amido black or Ponceau red stains (pp. 196, 206)
8. Absorbent paper
9. Acetic acid, 1 M

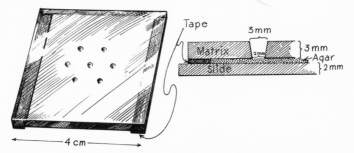

Fig. 1.2. Top view and cross-section of template for micro double-diffusion test (Wadsworth).

Method

1. Place the template on the agar-coated glass slide.
2. Fill a 1-ml pipette with warm agar (50-60°C), place the tip of the pipette near the open edge of the template, and allow the agar to run under the matrix in a continuous flow. With additional agar, seal the two open edges of the matrix. If in the process of filling the gel chamber the agar is forced up into the wells, it is advisable to remove some of it from the open side with a piece of absorbent paper so that the wells are of uniform size. If the agar has hardened and only one or two wells are filled, the agar can be carefully removed with a Pasteur pipette. The underlying agar layer should be left undisturbed.
3. Place the prepared plates in a humid chamber at room temperature, where they may be kept up to 30 minutes before filling.

4. Fill the wells using Pasteur pipettes. Tilt the pipette so that the reagent flows up into the pipette, leaving an air space in the bottom of the pipette. Place the tip of the pipette in the bottom of the well, and let the reagent run down into the well. If an air bubble forms, remove it and refill the well; otherwise, the bubble will prohibit the diffusion of the reagents.
5. Incubate the plates in a humid chamber one to three days at room temperature until precipitation lines appear.
6. Drawings may be made with the aid of oblique illumination without the removal of the matrix.
7. When the reaction is judged complete, the matrix is removed in the following way: a. The agar at the open sides of the chamber is cut away. b. The wells are rinsed with saline. c. The matrix is then slid off the agar, which adheres to the glass. d. A final record of the precipitation spectrum is made, and photographs may be taken.
8. Those plates that are not to be stored permanently are washed and stained with amido black or Ponceau red as previously described (p. 6).

REFERENCES

1. Barron, A. L. Reactions of viruses in agar gel. *Meth. in Virol. 5*, 347 (1971).
2. Ouchterlony, Ö. Diffusion-in-gel methods for immunological analysis. *Progr. Aller. 5*, 1 (1958).
3. ——————. *Handbook of Immunodiffusion and Immunoelectrophoresis* (Ann Arbor Science Publ.: Ann Arbor, Mich., 1968).
4. van Oss, C. J. Methods used in the characterization of immunoglobulins. In T. J. Greenwalt, Ed., *Advances in Immunogenetics* (Lippincott: Philadelphia, 1967).
5. ——————. Specifically impermeable precipitate, membranes formed through double diffusion in gels: Behavior with complex forming and with simple systems. *J. Coll. Inter. Sci. 27*, 684 (1968).
6. Wadsworth, C. A slide microtechnique for the analysis of immune precipitates in gel. *Int. Arch. Aller. Appl. Immunol. 10*, 355 (1957).
7. ——————. A microplate technique employing a gel chamber compared with other micro- and macroplate techniques for immune diffusion. *Int. Arch. Aller. Appl. Immunol. 21*, 131 (1962).

IMMUNOELECTROPHORESIS

Immunoelectrophoresis is a technique by which proteins are separated in an agar gel according to their surface charge, by exposing them to a direct-current electric field. After the electrophoretic separation, the proteins are allowed to react, by double-diffusion, with an antiserum deposited in a trough parallel to, and some distance away from, the newly spread-out proteins (Fig. 1.3).

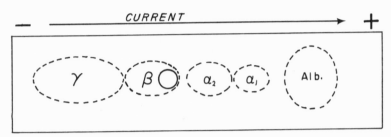

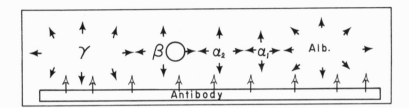

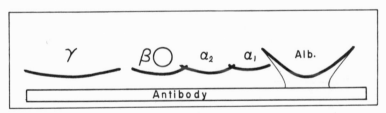

Fig. 1.3.

The result is a series of precipitate lines, generally in the form of more or less curved arcs (Fig. 1.4). Their formation obeys the laws described under "Gel Precipitation, Double-Diffusion" (p. 4), crossing of two lines indicating non-identity, fusing identity, and spurring partial identity. When a protein migrates electrophoretically in a very sharply defined homogeneous band (such as serum albumin), the resulting arc in immunoelectrophoresis will have the shape of a parabola. With an electrophoretically heterogeneous fraction (such as IgG), the precipitate arc will be a long line running almost parallel to the antiserum trough. Thus, abnormally homogeneous immunoglobulins, which occur in certain dysproteinemias, are easily recognizable by the shape of the precipitation arcs they produce in immunoelectrophoresis.

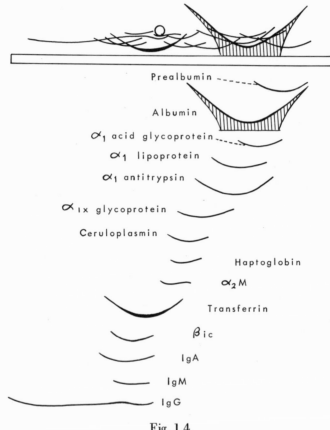

Prealbumin

Albumin

α_1 acid glycoprotein

α_1 lipoprotein

α_1 antitrypsin

α_{1x} glycoprotein

Ceruloplasmin

Haptoglobin

α_2 M

Transferrin

β_{ic}

IgA

IgM

IgG

Fig. 1.4.

Materials

1. Gel electrophoresis chamber
2. Micro-immunoelectrophoresis tray
3. Microscope slides (3 x 1 in.)
4. Filter paper wicks (8.5 x 2.5 in.)
5. Special agar, 1%, in barbital buffer (p. 208)
6. Barbital buffer, $\Gamma/2 = 0.05$, pH 8.2 (p. 196)
7. Pasteur pipettes and microliter pipettes.

Method

1. Fill electrophoresis chamber with barbital buffer, 700-800 ml; tilt to equalize liquid levels.
2. Line up slides on tray, place it on a level surface, and pipette hot agar onto tray. Gently try to press out any air bubbles trapped under the slides. Allow to harden 20-30 minutes.
3. Punch out pattern. Use suction pump fitted with Pasteur pipette or a special attachment to remove the agar from the wells. Use the appropriate knife to remove the agar from the troughs.
4. Apply samples to wells with capillary pipettes.
5. Place tray in chamber. Attach moist wicks over edges of the gel, and allow the other edge of the wicks to be in the buffer.
6. Subject to immunoelectrophoresis for four hours at 250 V, using at start 16-22 milliamperes (mA) and then increasing by about 10 mA.
7. Disconnect power supply, remove the tray, and fill the trough with the appropriate antiserum. Allow to react in moist chamber at room temperature overnight.
8. Results can be read, drawn, photographed and stained as previously described (p. 6).

REFERENCES

1. Arquembourg, P., Salvaggio, J. E., and Bickers, J. N. *Primer of Immuno-electrophoresis* (Ann Arbor-Humphrey Science Publ.: Ann Arbor, Mich.-London, 1970).
2. Grabar, P. and Burton, P. *Immuno-electrophoretic Analysis* (Elsevier: New York, 1964).
3. Williams, C. A. Immuno-electrophoretic analysis (IEA). In C. A. Williams and M. W. Chase, Eds., *Methods in Immunology and Immunochemistry*, vol. III (Academic: New York, 1971), p. 234.

QUANTITATIVE DETERMINATION OF SOLUBLE PROTEIN BY RADIAL DIFFUSION

The technique of single radial immunodiffusion was first developed for quantitative purposes by Mancini et al. and is based on the principle that when antigen has diffused from a cylindrical well into an agar gel in which its homologous antibody has been incorporated, a circular area of precipitation proportional to the antigen concentration forms around the well. Measurements are made of the diameters of precipitate rings formed by a series of known concentrations of antigen (standard solution) and of the unknown solutions placed on the plate. A plot of $\log_{10}$ concentration of known antigen (ordinate) versus diameter of precipitate ring (abscissa) should be a straight line, giving a standard curve from which the values of antigen concentrations in the unknown sample can be determined.

This method has been used to assay for immunoglobulin levels in patients' sera but can also be used to detect other soluble proteins. A so-called reversed variation of the method, wherein antigen is incorporated into the gel and wells are filled with its homologous antibody, has been used to quantitate antibodies.

Materials

1. Phosphate-buffered saline solution (PBS), pH 7.2
2. Special agar, 3% (p. 207)
3. Plastic petri dish with lid or glass slide
4. Tubular cutter for the wells (3-mm internal diameter)
5. Protein solution to be quantitated
6. Standard solution of protein being quantitated
7. Specific antiserum to protein being quantitated
8. Microliter pipettes

Method for Standardization of Antiserum

1. Melt special agar and keep in a 56°C waterbath
2. Prepare several dilutions of antiserum and warm to 56°C.
3. Mix equal volumes of melted agar with diluted antiserum and pour onto plate (or slide) so that the agar is approximately 1 mm thick. Prepare one plate for each antiserum dilution.
4. After the agar solidifies, punch six holes into agar and remove agar by suction.
5. Fill each hole to the top with dilutions of standard protein solution in the concentration range expected for unknowns. By filling the holes to the top rather than with a specific volume, compensation is made for variations in hole size caused by unevenness of plates.
6. Cover plates or place slides in a moist box for 24 hours at room temperature.
7. Examine plates and select antiserum concentrations that provide rings of optimum size.

Determination of Unknown Concentration

1. Prepare plates as above, using preselected antiserum solution.
2. Place twofold dilutions of standard protein solution into at least three holes.
3. Place twofold dilutions of unknown into three holes.
4. Allow diffusion to take place for 24 hours at room temperature.
5. Measure diameter of standard and unknown precipitation rings.
6. Plot standard curve and determine unknown concentrations.

REFERENCES

1. Fahey, J. L. and McKelvey, E. M. Quantitative determination of serum immunoglobulins in antibody-agar plates. *J. Immunol. 94*, 84 (1965).
2. Leikola, J. and Vyas, G. N. Human antibodies to ruminant IgM concealing the absence of IgA in man. *J. Lab. Clin. Med. 77*, 629 (1971).
3. Mancini, G., Carbonara, A. O., and Heremans, J. F. Immunochemical quantitation of antigens by single radial immunodiffusion. *Immunochem. 2*, 235 (1965).
4. Mancini, G., Vaerman, J. P., Carbonara, A. O., and Heremans, J. F. A single-radial-diffusion method for the immunological quantitation of proteins. *XI Colloquium on Protides of the Biological Fluids*. H. Peeter, ed. (Elsevier: Amsterdam, 1964), p. 370.
5. Stiehm, E. R. Radial diffusion technique for the quantitative estimation of precipitating antibody. *J. Lab. Clin. Med. 70*, 528 (1967).
6. Vaerman, J. P., Lebacq-Verheyden, A. M.. Scolari, L., and Heremans, J. F. Further studies on single radial immunodiffusion. I. Direct proportionality between area of precipitate and reciprocal of antibody concentration. II. The reversed system: diffusion of antibodies in antigen-containing gels. *Immunochem. 6*, 279, 287 (1969).

ELECTROIMMUNODIFFUSION

Electroimmunodiffusion, also known as single-diffusion one-dimensional electrophoresis or Laurell rocket immunoelectrophoresis, is a modification of the single-radial-diffusion method (Mancini technique) and uses an electrical current to force diffusion of the antigen in a gel containing antibody. Antigen reacts with antibody, giving precipitation zones like peaks (which Laurell has compared to "ascending rockets"; Fig. 1.5.). The distance between the top of the peak and the center of the well can be measured: at constant antibody concentrations, peak heights--or more precisely, the areas under the peaks--are proportional to the concentrations of the antigen.

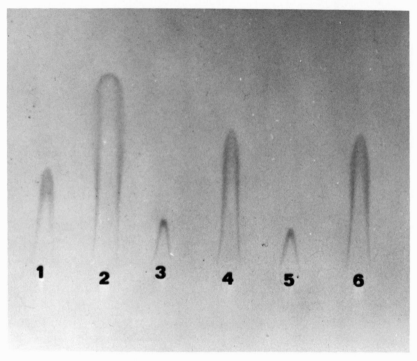

Fig. 1.5.

The technique is rapid, suitable for serial analysis, requires only small amounts of antigen (0.5-2.0 μg), and has been used for quantitative analysis of proteins, such as immunoglobulins, albumin, and thyroxin-binding globulin.

Materials

1. Special agar, 1%, in barbital buffer (p. 208)
2. Barbital buffer (p. 196)
3. Microliter pipette (5-10 μl)
4. Antigens, unknown and standard
5. Antiserum
6. Electrophoresis apparatus
7. Glass slides

Method

1. Mix desired amount of antiserum with special agar and pour on glass plate (see p. 12).
2. When agar has gelled, cut wells (3-3.5 mm in diameter along the line parallel with one of the long edges of the plate).
3. Fill wells with a measured amount of standard antigen or unknown antigen solution. Dilutions of standard antigen are used to obtain a standard curve.
4. Perform electrophoresis at 10V/cm for 2-10 hours, depending on the charge and amount of antigen applied in relation to antibody concentration.
5. Measure the height of the peaks directly under incident light. Alternatively, slides can be washed, dried, and stained as previously described (p. 6). After staining, measurements of peak heights are, of course, more accurate.

REFERENCES

1. Laurell, C. B. Quantitative estimation of proteins by electrophoresis in agarose gel containing antibodies. *Analyt. Biochem. 15*, 45 (1966).
2. Nielsen, H. G., Buus, O., and Weeke, B. A rapid determination of thyroxin-binding globulin in human serum by means of the Laurell rocket immuno-electrophoresis. *Clin. Chim. Acta 36*, 133 (1972).
3. Salvaggio, J. E., Arquembourg, P. C., and Gardnel, A. S. A comparison of the sensitivity of electroimmunodiffusion and single radial diffusion in quantitation of immunoglobulins in a dilute solution. *J. Aller. 46*, 326 (1970).
4. Watkins, J., Atkins, B., and Holborow, E. J. Quantitative estimation of protein by electroimmunodiffusion on Cellogel acetate membranes. *J. Clin. Pathol. 24*, 665 (1971).

QUANTITATIVE ONE-DIMENSIONAL
ENZYMOIMMUNOELECTROPHORESIS

The procedure of one-dimensional immunoelectrophoresis can be modified for use as a quantitative enzymal assay in the following manner:

1. An appropriate dilution of an antiserum to the enzyme is mixed with an equal volume of special agar. This dilution of antiserum must be chosen on the basis of experimental trials so that it is optimal for the resolution for the desired antigen-antibody systems. The antiserum-agar mixture is kept warm in a 55°C waterbath.
2. A glass plate (82 x 100 mm) is warmed by placing it on a Bunsen burner.

With a warmed serological pipette, 12.0 ml of the agar-antiserum mixture is poured onto the slide and allowed to gel. Pouring should be done with the slide on a warm leveling table. Once the agar has solidified, the plate is carefully transferred to the cold room for a few minutes.

3. Prepare and fill wells, and carry out electrophoresis as described for "Electroimmunodiffusion" (p. 15).
4. Immediately after the electrophoresis, the slide is placed in cold saline for one day at cold room temperature.
5. Apply the appropriate enzymatic stain.
6. Cover the slide with filter paper and air dry.
7. Determine the height or the areas of the stained peaks. Alternatively, they may be projected onto the white paper, traced, and cut out of the paper. Each peak is then weighed, with the weight of the peak being a reflection of the amount of enzyme present, compared with a standard run in the same plate.

ANTIGEN-ANTIBODY CROSSED ELECTROPHORESIS

Antigen-antibody crossed electrophoresis, also known as two-dimensional (Laurell) immunoelectrophoresis, was first proposed by Ressler and was later elaborated by Laurell. It attempts to obviate the fact that conventional immuno-electrophoresis is a qualitative technique, not suitable for quantitative evaluation of the different components identified. In this procedure different proteins are separated by electrophoresis in agar and then subjected to electrophoresis at a 90° angle in agar containing antibodies to the different proteins (Fig. 1.6.).

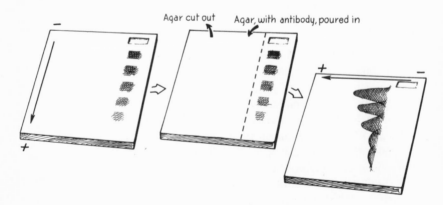

Fig. 1.6.

Because of the rapidity with which antigen and antibody meet, the reaction is concluded in a very short time, and because of the direction of the second electrophoresis, precipitation bands are not superimposed but rather appear as peaks that are separated in relation to the mobility of the various proteins. Again, as in the Mancini technique, the areas of the precipitate peaks are proportional to the concentrations of the antigens that formed them.

The antigen-antibody crossed electrophoresis has been used mostly to detect levels of various plasma proteins in pathological conditions but can also be applied to all the other proteins that can be studied by conventional immunoelectrophoresis.

Materials

1. Special agar, 1%, in barbital buffer (p. 208)
2. Barbital buffer pH 8.2, $\Gamma/2 = 0.05$ (p. 196)
3. Human serum
4. Rabbit or goat antiserum to whole human serum
5. Electrophoresis apparatus
6. Microliter pipettes
7. Phosphate-buffered saline solution (PBS), pH 7.2
8. Glass slides (8.3 x 10.2 cm)

Method

1. Pour twelve ml of special agar onto a glass slide on a leveling table. After the agar solidifies, cut a well using a cutter 0.8x0.2 cm. This well must be 2 cm from the cathodal end and 2.2 cm from the edge.
2. Dilute the normal human serum (or antigen) with barbital buffer. Mix it with an equal volume of special agar, fill the antigen well with the antigen-agar mixture and seal with a drop of agar.
3. Subject the plate to electrophoresis for two and a half hours at room temperature in a humidified chamber. In this electrophoresis, 40V are employed. Paper wicks and barbital buffer are used as described for "Immunoelectrophoresis" (p. 11).
4. After the run is completed, cut away the agar layer to the left of the antigen well. (This is approximately 5.5 x 10.2 cm in area.) Replace it with 8 ml of special agar containing antiserum diluted in barbital buffer. After the layer solidifies, seal the cut with agar containing no serum. The dilutions of the antigen and the antiserum have to be predetermined experimentally.
5. Put fresh barbital buffer in the electrophoresis chambers, and perform a

second electrophoresis run at 40V, with the cathodal end being nearest the antigen, for one or one and a half hours at room temperature.

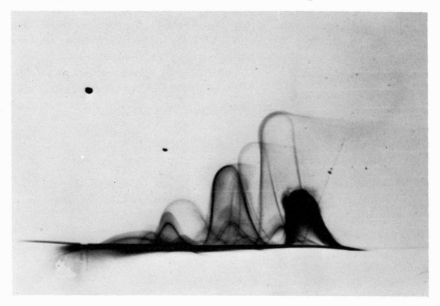

Fig. 1.7.

6. After electrophoresis wash the plate immediately in PBS for two days at room temperature. Air dry and stain with Ponceau red or other protein stains (p. 6).
7. The areas of the stained peaks (Fig. 1.7) may be measured by planimetry. Alternatively, they may be projected onto white paper, traced, and cut out. Each area is then weighed, with the weight of the area being a reflection of the amount of antigen present compared with a standard.

REFERENCES

1. Laurell, C. B. Antigen-antibody crossed electrophoresis. *Analyt. Biochem.* *10*, 358 (1965).
2. Minchin Clarke, H. G. Two-dimensional (Laurell) immunoelectrophoresis for estimation of antigens in relative units. In C. A. Williams and M. W. Chase, Eds., *Methods in Immunology and Immunochemistry*, vol. III (Academic: New York, 1971), p. 287.
3. Ressler, N. Two-dimensional electrophoresis of protein antigens with an antibody containing buffer. *Clin. Chim. Acta 5*, 795 (1960).

COUNTERIMMUNOELECTROPHORESIS

Counterimmunoelectrophoresis, also known as crossover electrophoresis or immunoelectroosmophoresis (IEOP), makes use of the endosmotic flow, which during electrophoresis causes the slow moving γ globulins to be displaced toward the cathode. In this manner the antibodies move as a concentrated front toward the cathode, while the antigens move in the opposite direction toward the anode. By appropriate arrangement of wells, antibody and antigen can thus be made to converge, resulting in the formation of a precipitate between the two wells. The precipitation lines develop rapidly and usually reach maximum intensity in this system within 30 to 90 minutes, depending upon the strength of the reagents.

This technique is currently being used for the detection of hepatitis-associated (Australia) antigen (HAA) in serum of patients with viral hepatitis and in donor blood prior to transfusion. Such a screening test for HAA on blood before transfusion is now required by law in many states.

Note: It is now known that serum hepatitis may be transmitted by both parenteral and oral routes. Since studies have indicated that HAA may be the causative agent of serum hepatitis or at least may be carried in close association with the infectious agent, the following precautions are recommended when performing the test:

(1)   The test should be carried out in an isolated area, preferably under a biological safety hood.

(2)   No mouth pipetting should be performed in this area. An automatic pipetting device should be used if any dilutions are required.

(3)   Disposable gloves, a face mask, and a laboratory coat should be worn when working in this area. Gloves should be considered contaminated after use. When handling instruments outside the immediate working area, such as the IEOP cell or power supply, the gloves should be changed.

(4)   A disinfectant, such as 10% formalin, should be available to clean the working area.

(5)   All contaminated materials should be disposed of either in a plastic bag for incinerating or in a closed stainless-steel container for autoclaving.

Materials

1.   Sera under examination for HAA

2.   HAA-positive control sera (a strongly positive and a weakly positive control)
3.   HAA-negative control sera
4.   Antibody to HAA (anti-HAA)
5.   Barbital buffer, pH 8.2, $\Gamma/2 = 0.05$ (p. 196)
6.   Special agar, 1%, in barbital buffer (p. 208)
7.   Pasteur pipettes
8.   Power supply and IEOP cell (two troughs with electrodes in a moisturized chamber)
9.   Glass slides, 3.25 x 4 in.

Method

1.   Prepare an even layer of 1% special agar on a glass slide by placing the slide on a leveling table and slowly pipetting 15 ml of the agar-barbital solution over the slide. The agar is evenly distributed on the slide by carefully spreading it over the glass surface with the pipette tip. Once the agar has solidified, the plates are stored in a humidified chamber at 4°C.

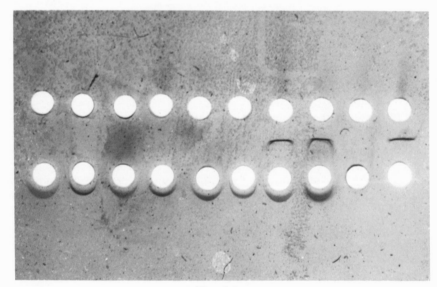

Fig. 1.8.

2.   Cut wells for antigen and antibody using the template provided (Fig. 1.8). Each well is 3 mm in diameter, with 5 mm between the antigen and antibody well (edge to edge). A plate of this size will accommodate two sets

of antibody-antigen rows. Notice that the antibody wells are always oriented on the anodal side in each set of the horizontal rows, while the patient's
serum or antigen control is placed in the wells on the cathodal side of the
horizontal row (Fig. 1.9).

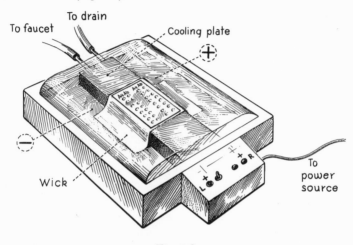

Fig. 1.9.

3. Using a Pasteur pipette, fill the wells. Enough reagent is added until the
    wells are completely filled. A separate disposable pipette is used for each
    patient's serum. Each plate contains three controls: HAA-negative control
    serum, a strongly HAA-positive control serum, and a weakly HAA-positive
    control serum.
4. Before starting the electrophoresis, start circulating water through the
    cooling unit between the two buffer troughs of the electrophoretic cell.
5. As soon as all the wells have been filled, the plate is positioned on the
    cooling unit so that the date inscribed on the glass plate is on the anodal
    side. In this position, the antibody wells are toward the anode, while the
    antigen wells are cathodally oriented.
6. Place filter wicks (6 x 4.5 cm) folded lengthwise across the anodal and
    cathodal ends of the plate, while the other ends of the paper wicks are
    immersed in the buffer. Care should be taken to insure that air bubbles are
    not trapped in the double folded lengths of filter paper. The filter paper
    should be saturated with buffer. One end of the filter paper wick is
    positioned over the agar plate to provide an overlap of approximately 0.5
    in. (1 cm).
7. Electrophoresis should be carried out for 90 minutes at a terminal voltage
    of 200V. Milliamperage at 200V is approximately 30 mA per plate: it

should not exceed 50. The temperature of the cell should be approximately 15°C. After the electrophoresis the wicks are treated and disposed of as contaminated material.

8.   Examine the plate for precipitation lines at the end of the 90-minute period. The plate should be considered contaminated and precautions should be taken during its handling after electrophoresis. When high-titered sera (HAA-positive at a titer greater than 64) are subjected to electrophoresis for a long period, a false negative reaction may occur. These sera usually exhibit a positive reaction early during the electrophoresis period and later become negative because of the antigen excess that results during continued electrophoresis. For this reason, in some laboratories plates are examined periodically during electrophoresis. This is advisable if it can be performed without an interruption in the electrophoretic separation. Because of the problem of the false negative reactions in antigen excess, a high-titered serum should be incorporated into the test as one of the positive controls.

After electrophoresis the results for each serum are noted, the plate is placed in a humidified chamber, and a second reading is made 30-60 minutes later. A precipitation line between the antigen and antibody wells is indicative of a positive reaction. If a precipitin line appears to be positioned abnormally to the wells, the specimen should be retested using both a diluted (1:5 with buffer) and undiluted serum sample.

Although it is possible to wash, dry, and stain the plate so that a permanent record may be kept, we regard the plate as contaminated and prefer not to carry out this procedure. The reactions are noted on the protocol sheet, and the plates are discarded in a bath of 10% formalin and eventually disposed of by incineration. However, if a permanent record is desired, the plates may be washed in isotonic saline. Changing the wash bath two or three times a day for two days is sufficient for washing. It has been our practice to soak the plate in a bath of 10% formalin before drying. The plates are air-dried after placing a wet piece of filter paper over the agarose. After drying, the plates may be stained with one of the protein stains as indicated in the section on "Reagents" (pp. 196, 206).

All specimens positive for HAA by IEOP should be tested in double diffusion with known HAA-positive control serum to confirm the IEOP results.

REFERENCES

1.   Blumberg, B. S., Sutnick, A. I., and London, W. T. Australia antigen as a hepatitis virus. *Am. J. Med.* 48, 1 (1970).

2.   Bull. WHO. Viral hepatitis and tests for the Australia (hepatitis-associated) antigen and antibody. *42*, 957 (1970).
3.   Hansson, B. G., Kidnmark, C. O., and Johnsson, T. Comparison between the immunoelectroosmophoresis and Ouchterlony precipitation technique in detecting Australia antigen in cases of hepatitis. *Vox Sang. 19*, 225 (1970).
4.   Prince, A. M. and Burke, K. Serum hepatitis antigen (SH): Rapid selection by high voltage immunoelectroosmophoresis. *Science 169*, 593 (1970).
5.   Prince, A. M., Hargrove, R. L., Szumness, W., Cherubin, C. E., Fontana, V. J., and Jefties, G. H. Immunologic distinction between infectious and serum hepatitis. *N. E. J. Med. 282*, 987 (1970).
6.   Sutnick, A., London, W. T., Millman, I., Coyne, V., and Blumberg, B. Viral hepatitis. *Med. Clinics of N. A. 54*, 805 (1970).
7.   Sutnick, A. I., London, W. T., Millman, I., Gerstley, B. J. S., and Blumberg, B. Ergasteric hepatitis: Endemic hepatitis associated with Australia antigen in a research laboratory. *Ann. Int. Med. 75*, 35 (1971).

IMMUNORHEOPHORESIS

In the conventional double-diffusion immunoprecipitation reaction, where the reagents are brought together by molecular diffusion, only a small portion of both reagents will diffuse toward one another. Most of the reagents diffuse away from one another in various directions and never meet. This is a major cause of the relatively low sensitivity of this type of reaction.

The efficiency of the reaction can be improved if a higher proportion of the two reagents can be brought together. This can be done by electrophoretic transport, but only in cases where the antigen and antibody have significantly different isoelectric pH's and only after careful selection of a buffer with a pH intermediate between these two. Another method of bringing the reagents together is by hydrodynamic transport. This method can be applied at any pH and without regard to whether antigen and antibody have different isoelectric points. In all cases an approximately threefold increase in efficiency is obtained, resulting in a threefold increase in sensitivity.

The method works as follows: hydrodynamic transport of antigen as well as antibody from their respective wells toward one another is obtained through the continuous evaporation of water from the gel above the spot where the precipitation reaction is to take place. If enough extra buffer is provided at the periphery, it flows continuously into the gel by capillary action toward the place where the evaporation is taking place, thus bringing antigen and antibody together (Fig. 1.10).

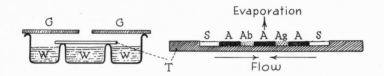

Fig. 1.10. Schematic drawing of apparatus for unidimensional immunorheophoresis. A: agar; Ab: antibody well filled with antiserum; Ag: antigen well filled with antigen solution; S: solution; T: carrier tray; W: water; G: glass plates serving as cover, arranged so that the evaporation slit is left open above the middle of the agar plate.

Materials

1. Phosphate-buffered saline solution (PBS), pH 7.2 (p. 205)
2. Human serum albumin (HSA) (0.1% in PBS)
3. Rabbit antiserum to human serum albumin
4. Special agar, 0.5%, with 1% glycerol
5. 0.05 M NaCl, 1% glycerol solution
6. Plastic immunoelectrophoresis trays
7. Metal punch (5 mm diameter)
8. Electrophoresis chamber
9. Glass plates
10. Pasteur pipettes

Method

1. Cast in a tray a 1.5 mm thick layer of special agar dissolved in a watery solution of 0.05 M sodium chloride and 1.0% glycerol (the glycerol is needed to keep the gel from drying out). The salt concentration of 0.05 M is chosen so that a slight local increase in ionic strength close to the place of strongest evaporation will not create any disturbing effects. In practice the average increase in salt concentration in that place is no more than 15%, while the highest increase encountered remains under 25%. The greater increase in protein concentration than in salt concentration between the wells is undoubtedly caused by the very low diffusivity of protein as compared to small ions. Plastic immunoelectrophoresis trays may be used, with the holes taped up.
2. After setting, punch wells of 5-mm diameter 4 mm apart and then remove a 2.5-cm-wide band of agar at both edges. The space obtained is filled with the solution of 0.05 M sodium chloride and 1% glycerol. The wells are filled with antigen and antibody solutions (Ag and Ab). The bottom of the tank

is filled to a height of 1-2 cm with water (to assure a high degree of humidity in the tank), and the tank is covered with two glass plates 9 mm above the gel surface, leaving an open slit 9 mm wide. The edges of the glass plates are exactly above the centers of the Ag and Ab wells. The precipitate is allowed to form overnight.

REFERENCE

1.   van Oss, C. J. and Bronson, P. M. Immunorheophoresis. *Immunochem. 6*, 775 (1969).

ENZYMOIMMUNOELECTROPHORESIS

Enzymoelectrophoresis and enzymoimmunoelectrophoresis are performed like simple electrophoresis and immunoelectrophoresis. The main difference is in the staining procedure. Rather than using a protein stain such as amido black or Ponceau red, selective stains for enzymes are employed. This method allows for the detection and identification of proteins with enzymatic activity. Since the enzymatic activity of many proteins is retained after uniting with antibody, the staining procedure is applicable after either electrophoresis or immunoelectrophoresis. As a rule, staining reactions are carried out immediately following enzymoelectrophoresis. However, in the case of enzymoimmunoelectrophoresis, after the development of the precipitation pattern, the plates are washed for three or four days and dried prior to staining. Agarose has been found to be superior to agar as a matrix for the testing of the enzymes, because impurities often found in the agar may inhibit or minimize some staining reactions. An advantage of such a staining technique resides in increasing the sensitivity for detecting an immunological reaction. A relatively small amount of enzyme in an antibody-antigen complex reacts during the staining procedure to amplify the immunological reaction. Enzymoimmunoelectrophoresis is a very sensitive assay and provides for the immunologic and enzymatic characterization of proteins.

Materials

1.   Esterase staining
     A.   Indoxyl acetate solution (p. 198) prepared immediately before use
     B.   β-naphthyl acetate-diazonium salt solution (p. 198)
     C.   1M acetic acid

2. Catalase staining
   A. Hydrogen peroxide (3% for first method, 0.1% for second method)
   B. 4.0% potassium iodide*
   C. 4.0% starch in barbital buffer, pH 7.4*
   D. 0.2M acetic acid*
   *B, C, and D are used only in the second method

Method

1. Esterase staining
   A. Using indoxyl acetate
      (1) Immerse the slide in the indoxyl acetate solution and incubate for several hours (4-12 hours).
      (2) Decolorize with 2% acetic acid until the background is clear. Esterase hydrolyzes the ester bond producing free indoxyl. The indoxyl is oxidized in air to produce insoluble blue indigo. Cupric acetate facilitates the oxidation procedure. Esterase-active areas or precipitation arcs possessing esterase appear as a deep blue color.
   B. Using β-naphthyl acetate
      (1) Immerse the plate in the β-naphthyl acetate-diazonium salt solution and incubate it from one to three hours.
      (2) Decolorize the plates with 2% acetic acid until the background is clear. The esterase releases free β-naphthol from the substrate (β-naphthyl acetate). The β-naphthol then combines with the diazonium salt (diazo blue B). This combination results in a purple, insoluble complex which localizes the esterase.
2. Catalase staining (Catalase activity is resolved best after immunoelectrophoresis if the plates are not dried.)
   A. Using hydrogen peroxide
      Immerse the plate for 10-20 minutes in 3% hydrogen peroxide. Catalase-active areas are delineated by the evolution of bubbles. Oxygen is released from the substrate, hydrogen peroxide by the catalytic activity of the enzyme.
   B. Using starch and hydrogen peroxide
      (1) Immerse the plate for 10 minutes in a solution containing equal volumes of 4% starch and 0.1% hydrogen peroxide.
      (2) Pour off solution. Wait 10-15 minutes. Rinse the plate a few seconds in tap water.
      (3) Immerse the plate in a solution containing 4% potassium iodide (acidified with a few drops of 0.2M acetic acid).

(4)   When the background of the agarose has become blue, the plate is removed and blotted dry with filter paper.

In the second method, hydrogen peroxide also serves as the substrate for catalase. In the presence of hydrogen peroxide, iodine is liberated from potassium iodide. The iodine combines with the starch entrapped in the agarose to give a blue-black color. In the areas containing catalase, the hydrogen peroxide has been enzymatically cleaved and is not available to release free iodine from the potassium iodide. Catalase activity is visualized as a clear area in the purple-blue background.

REFERENCES

1.   Bartholomew, E., Bartholomew, W. R., and Rose, N. R. Isoenzyme differences between a human diploid cell line, Wl-38 and SV_{40} transformed Wl-38. *J. Immunol. 103*, 787 (1969).

2.   Bartholomew, W. R. Multiple catalase enzymes in two species of Mycobacterium. *Am. Rev. Resp. Dis. 97*, 710 (1968).

3.   Bartholomew, W. R., Bartholomew, E., Knowles, B. B., and Rose, N. R. Immunochemical detection of a human species-specific esterase in interspecies hybrid cells. *Exp. Cell Res. 70*, 376 (1971).

4.   Therrien, G. D., Rose, N. R., and Bartholomew, W. R. Purification and characterization of a human-specific esterase from urine. *Prep. Biochem. 1*, 259 (1971).

5.   Uriel, J. Characterization of enzymes in specific immunoprecipitates. *Ann. N. Y. Acad. Sci. 103*, 956 (1963).

6.   ——————. Color reactions for the identification of antigen-antibody precipitates in gels. In C. A. Williams and M. W. Chase, Eds., *Methods in Immunology and Immunochemistry*, vol. III (Academic: New York, 1971), p. 294.

AUTORADIOGRAPHY OF PRECIPITATION REACTIONS IN GEL

When either antigen or antibody has been radio-labeled and they interact in immunoelectrophoresis, double-diffusion gel precipitation or single immunodiffusion, the reaction (visible to the naked eye or invisible) can be confirmed by exposing a special X-ray film to the agar plate or slide. This kind of autoradiography is very helpful in detecting antibody activity (associated with single or multiple immunoglobulins) in serum or other body fluids consisting of many protein components.

Two methods have been described:

One-Step Procedure

Antiserum to a particular antigen (e.g., to human IgG) is mixed with radio-labeled antigen to which antibody is expected. Both react simultaneously against, for example, whole serum examined for the presence of antibodies.

Two-Step Procedure

Antigen and antibody are diffused in agar gel and after completion of the diffusion and extensive washing to remove free proteins, either radio-labeled antigen or antibody is added to the appropriate well. The labeled antigen (or antibody) diffuses and precipitates with its antibody (or antigen) and the precipitation line will be demonstrated by autoradiography. This procedure can be applied to all reactions in gel, such as double diffusion, single radial diffusion, or immunoelectrophoresis. Small quantities of IgE (as little as 20 ng) have been detected by this technique in single radial immunodiffusion using radio-labeled antiserum.

Double-diffusion gel precipitation (also known as radioimmunodiffusion, or RID)

Materials

1. Labeled antigen (For other reagents, see double-diffusion gel precipitation, p. 5)
2. X-ray film, Kodak, Kk
3. Developer, Bauman-Diafine two-bath developer, A & B

Method

1. Perform double-diffusion gel precipitation on plate or microscopic slide (p. 5).
2. After extensive washing in borate buffer for 24 hours (change the buffer several times), rinse the wells with distilled water and thoroughly dry wells with filter paper.
3. Add labeled antigen to the antigen well and incubate for 24 hours in moist chamber at room temperature.

4. Wash again in borate buffer for 24 hours. Rinse wells with distilled water. Dry slides using wet filter paper and fan.
5. When slides are completely dry, expose X-ray film to them for three days and develop the film.
6. Dried slides can be stained with amido black stain.
7. Compare the precipitation pattern (stained slide) with the X-ray pattern.

Immunoelectrophoresis (also known as radioimmunoelectrophoresis, or RIE)

Materials

1. Labeled antigen (For other reagents, see under immunoelectrophoresis, p. 10)
2. X-ray film, Kodak, Kk
3. Developer, Bauman-Diafine two-bath developer, A & B

Method

1. Perform immunoelectrophoresis as previously described (p. 11).
2. After washing in borate buffer for 24 hours, rinse the wells and trough with distilled water; thoroughly dry wells and trough with filter paper.
3. Add labeled antigen to the trough and incubate for 24 hours in moist chamber at room temperature. The antigen, if necessary, can be diluted. As diluent, serum of the same species as the antiserum applied is used; in most cases it is normal rabbit serum or normal goat serum diluted 1:30.
4. Wash again in borate buffer for 24 hours. Rinse wells and trough with distilled water. Cover slides with wet filter paper and dry them using a fan.
5. When slides are completely dry, expose X-ray film to them for three to four days (or longer) and develop the film. The time of developing depends on the activity of the labeled compound.
6. Stain slides three to five minutes in amido black stain. Rinse with water and destain in destaining solution. Rinse with distilled water and dry for a few minutes under fan. Coat with protective spray and mount on plexiglass or cardboard.
7. Compare the precipitation pattern of the stained slide with the pattern on the X-ray film.

REFERENCES

1. Arbesman, C. E., Ito, K., Wypych, J., and Wicher, K. One step single radial diffusion method using ^{125}I labeled antiserum for the determination of IgE levels. *J. Aller. 47*, 85 (1971).
2. Rowe, D. S. Radioactive single radial diffusion. *Bull. WHO 40*, 613 (1969).
3. Thorbecke, G. J., Hochwald, G. M., and Williams, C. A. Autoradiography of antigen-antibody reactions in gels. In C. A. Williams and M. W. Chase, Eds., *Methods in Immunology and Immunochemistry*, vol. III (Academic: New York, 1971), p. 343.
4. Yagi, Y. Identification of multiple antibody components by radioimmuno-electrophoresis and radioimmunodiffusion. In C. A. Williams and M. W. Chase, Eds., *Methods in Immunology and Immunochemistry*, vol. III (Academic: New York, 1971), p. 463.
5. Yagi, Y., Maier, P., and Pressman, D. Immunoelectrophoretic identification of guinea pig anti-insulin antibodies. *J. Immunol. 89*, 736 (1962).
6. Yagi, Y., Maier, P., Pressman, D., Arbesman, C. E., and Reisman, R. E. The presence of the ragweed-binding antibodies in the β2A, β2M, and γ globulins of the sensitive individual. *J. Immunol. 91*, 83 (1963).

Chapter 2

COMPLEMENT DETERMINATIONS

N. Rose   W. Bartholomew
P. Bigazzi   R. Zarco

Complement is a system of serum factors that is activated by an immune complex and that, in turn, mediates various biological phenomena. Partial or complete activation can also be caused by aggregated γ globulin, cobra venom, tissue protease, certain lysosomal enzymes, trypsin, plasmin, and endotoxin. The

Table 2.1.   WHO Nomenclature of Complement Components (1968)

Recommended Nomenclature for Complement Components		Previous Designation	Approximate Electrophoretic Mobility (Human C)	Approximate Sedimentation Coefficient (Svedberg units; Human C)
C1	C1q	11S component, $C'0$	$\gamma2$	11
	C1r		β	7
	C1s	C'1-esterase (after activation)	$\alpha2$	4
C4		β1E globulin	$\beta1$	10
C2			$\beta2$	6
C3		C'3c, C'3a, β1C globulin	$\beta1$	10
C5		C'3b, β1F globulin	$\beta1$	8.7
C6		C'3e, C'3α	$\beta2$	6
C7		C'3f, C'3β	$\beta2$	6
C8		C'3a, C'3c	$\gamma1$	8
C9		C'3d	$\alpha2$	5

successive stages of complement activation have been most studied using the reaction of immune hemolysis, which occurs when red blood cells are treated with antibody and complement. The terminology now in use is based on the hemolytic sequence, and the nine components of complement are designated with the letter "C" and a number (Table 2.1).

The complement sequence in immune hemolysis and the substances and biological phenomena mediated by complement are outlined in Fig. 2.1. A kininlike substance has been isolated that may be a product of C2; anaphylotoxins may derive from C3 and C5; chemotactic factors may arise from C5 and C6,7. The binding of C3 and C4 to the immune complex conditions immune adherence, a phenomenon related to the enhancement of phagocytosis, also mediated by the binding of C3. Membrane damage seems to be caused by C8, but lysis is greatly accelerated by C9.

The binding of complement in the immune hemolytic reaction is utilized in the complement fixation test, which for years has been used for qualitative and quantitative studies in microbiology and immunology. Antibodies against different bacteria and viruses or against several tissue antigens as well as antigens of microorganisms or tissues can be detected by this sensitive technique.

Variations in the levels of total complement activity or of some of the individual components of complement have been observed in certain human diseases, and the evaluation of such changes can be helpful both in the diagnosis and the treatment of these pathological conditions.

REFERENCES

1.   Alpen, C. A. and Rosen, F. S. Genetic aspects of the complement system. *Advances in Immunol. 14*, 251 (1971).
2.   Bruninga, G. L. Complement--A review of the chemistry and reaction mechanisms. *Am. J. Clin. Pathol. 55*, 273 (1971).
3.   Nomenclature of Complement. *WHO Bull. 39*, 935 (1968)
4.   Cooper, R. N., Polley, M. J. and Müller-Eberhard, H. J. Biology of complement. In M. Samter, Ed., *Immunological Diseases* (Little, Brown: Boston, 1971), p. 289.
5.   Rapp, H. J. and Borsos, T. *Molecular Basis of Complement Action* (Appleton-Century Crofts: New York, 1970).
6.   Ruddy, S., Gigli, I., and Austen, K. F. The complement system of man. *New Engl. J. Med. 287*, 489 (1972).

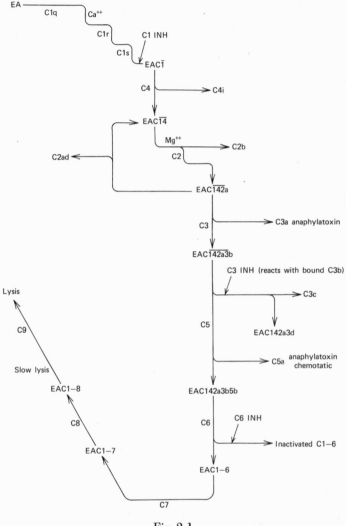

Fig. 2.1.

COMPLEMENT FIXATION TEST

The complement fixation test represents a sensitive technique for the measurement of antibody or antigen. Since each antibody molecule may trigger the activation of hundreds of complement molecules, a considerable amplification of the antigen-antibody reaction can be achieved.

Many modifications of this technique have been devised, but generally all are performed in two stages. In the first, antigen-antibody mixtures are incubated with a measured amount of complement; in the second, a suspension of sheep red blood cells (SRBC or E) sensitized with anti-SRBC rabbit hemolysin (amboceptor or A) is added to the mixture as an indicator system to detect free (unfixed) complement after the original antigen-antibody reaction.

Complement can be measured most accurately by determining the quantity necessary to hemolyze 50% of a standard suspension of sensitized red blood cells. A quantitative test can be performed by measuring the actual number of 50% hemolytic units (CH_{50}) of complement fixed at the optimal ratio of antibody and antigen. A common practice in the clinical diagnostic laboratory is to measure the dilution of patient's serum able to give 50% fixation of a standard quantity of complement using a previously determined optimal dilution of antigen. Controls must be included to detect anticomplementary (or procomplementary) effects of antigen and antiserum.

Two methods will be described, the main difference between them being the use of small amounts of reagents in the second, in which a special plate with small wells is employed instead of tubes. As examples of the variation in methodology commonly employed, the first method starts with a somewhat arbitrary dilution of complement and regulates the hemolytic reaction by subsequent titration of amboceptor. In the second method, complement is predetermined accurately and amboceptor is employed at an arbitrary (although plateau) dilution. The buffers used as diluents also differ, although either buffer may be used for either test.

Macromethod

In the following simplified procedure an arbitrarily selected dilution of complement is prepared and part of it is mixed with antigen and antibody. The next day a titration of the amboceptor is performed using the remaining part of the complement dilution prepared the previous day. The amboceptor dilution optimal for the concentration of complement used the previous day is selected to sensitize red cells. Then the sensitized red blood cells are added to the mixture of antigen, antibody, and complement prepared the first day.

Materials

1. Bovine serum albumin (BSA) solution, 0.05 $\mu g/ml$
2. Anti-BSA rabbit serum, inactivated at $56°C$ for 30 minutes to destroy complement
3. Pooled guinea pig complement

4. Rabbit antiserum to SRBC or SRBC stroma (amboceptor), 50% glycer-
    inated
5. SRBC
6. Triethanolamine buffered saline (TEAE) (p. 209)
7. Test tubes, 12 x 75 mm
8. Pipettes, 1 ml

Method

1. Dilute inactivated antiserum in two rows of nine tubes each, using twofold
    serial dilutions (volume 0.1 ml), starting with a 1:10 dilution. To a control
    tube in each row add 0.1 ml buffer.
2. To each tube in the first row (including the control tube) add 0.1 ml of
    BSA solution. Add 0.1 ml buffer to each tube in the second row.
3. Add 0.1 ml of guinea pig complement to every tube in the test. Shake well.
    The commercial complement is diluted 1:15. Retain 1.8 ml of the same
    complement dilution to make amboceptor titration on the following day.
4. Incubate test overnight at 4°C. Keep complement sample at 4°C.

Protocol 2.1.   Complement Fixation Test

| | | Hemolysis | |
Tube	Antiserum Dilution	BSA	TEAE
1	1:10		
2	1:20		
3	1:40		
4	1:80		
5	1:160		
6	1:320		
7	1:640		
8	1:1280		
9	1:2560		
10	control		

Note: *The following steps will be performed on second day.*

5.   On following day, wash sheep red blood cells three times in buffer and make a 4% suspension.
6.   Make an amboceptor titration as follows, using buffer, the complement sample, and the amboceptor diluted 1:400:

Protocol 2.2.   Amboceptor Titration

Tube no.	Buffer ml	Amboceptor	Dilution of amboceptor
A	2.8	0.2	1:6000
B	1.5	0.5 of Tube A	1:24,000
		From Tube A	
1	0	0.6	1:6000
2	0.2	0.4	1:9000
3	0.3	0.3	1:12,000
4	0.4	0.2	1:18,000
		From Tube B	
5	0	0.6	1:24,000
6	0.2	0.4	1:36,000
7	0.3	0.3	1:48,000
8	0.4	0.2	1:72,000
9	0.5	0	none

Add 0.2 ml complement to tubes 1-9.
Add 0.2 ml 4% sheep cells to tubes 1-9.
7.   Take main test out of refrigerator and incubate for one hour at 37°C.
8.   Incubate amboceptor titration 30 minutes at 37°C. Determine the dilution of amboceptor necessary to give approximately 2.5 hemolytic units (i.e., 2.5 times the greatest dilution providing complete hemolysis). Mix equal volume of 4% sheep erythrocytes with diluted amboceptor. Incubate with swirling for 5 minutes at 37°C.
9.   After the main test has incubated a total of one hour at 37°C, add 0.2 ml of the sensitized cells to each tube in the test. Shake well.

10. Incubate test again at $37°C$ for 10-15 minutes or until the controls are lysed; take the first reading. After an additional incubation period of 20 minutes at $37°C$, take the second reading. A third reading is taken after two hours incubation at $37°C$.

Approximate the extent of lysis visually as follows:

−	complete lysis
+	almost complete lysis
++	50% lysis
+++	trace of lysis
++++	no lysis

Micromethod

Materials

1. Inactivated rabbit antiserum (diluted 1:100) to hen egg albumin
2. Dilutions of crystalline hen egg albumin (Pentex) in normal saline solution, labeled A, B, C, D, and E.
3. Guinea pig complement serum yielding 4 CH_{50} units per milliliter (Consult p. 40 for the standard method of determining CH_{50}.)
4. Sheep erythrocytes sensitized with 1:2000 rabbit antibody against SRBC (EA), 1×10^8 cells per milliliter
5. Veronal buffered saline (p. 209)
6. V-shaped microliter plates
7. Pasteur pipettes, droppers and diluters

Method

1. Label a V-shaped microtiter plate alongside of the plate starting with 100 on top of the first well and twofold increasing numbers, 200-102,400, on top of second to eleventh wells. Label the rows along the short side of the plate A, B, C, D, E, and F.
2. Using a dropper, place a drop of buffer into the second to the twelfth wells of rows A-F.
3. With a Pasteur pipette, place two drops of antibody 1:100, into the first wells of rows A-F. With the microtiter diluter, loop out a serial twofold dilution from the first well to the eleventh well of each row.
4. Using separate droppers for each dilution of antigen, add one drop into the wells of the corresponding rows A-E.
5. Place one drop of buffer into each well of row F and in the twelfth well of rows A-F.

6. Add one drop of guinea pig complement into all wells. Incubate the plate at 4°C overnight using a cover over the wells to prevent evaporation of reaction mixture.
7. After the overnight incubation, transfer the plate into a 37°C incubator and incubate for 30 minutes.
8. Add one drop of EA suspension into all wells and incubate the plate at 37°C for 60 minutes.
9. Centrifuge the plate to sediment non-lysed cells at 1000 rpm for 5 minutes.
10. Determine the degree of lysis by noting the size of the button of intact cells and the color of the supernatant. The titer for each dilution of antigen is the highest dilution of antiserum allowing 50% lysis of the SRBC.

REFERENCES

1. Kabat, E. A. and Mayer, M. M. *Experimental Immunochemistry* (Thomas: Springfield, Ill., 1961).
2. Kite, J. H., Brown, R. C., and Rose, N. R. Autoantibodies to thyroid tissue sediment detected by the antiglobulin consumption test. *J. Lab. Clin. Med.* *59*, 179 (1962).
3. Reichlin, M. Complement fixation. In N. R. Rose, F. Milgrom, and C. J. van Oss, Eds., *Principles of Immunology* (Macmillan Co., in press).
4. Witebsky, E., Rose, N. R., and Shulman, S. Studies on organ specificity. I. The serological specificity of thyroid extracts. *J. Immunol.* *75*, 269 (1955).

COMPLEMENT ACTIVITY IN HUMAN DISEASE

Elevated complement levels have been observed in sera from patients with acute myocardial infarction, dermatomyositis, periarteritis nodosa, acute rheumatic fever, acute polyarthritis, thyroiditis, and other inflammatory diseases or in some stages of serum sickness.

Lower complement levels or decreases or absence of components of the complement systems have been detected in a variety of hereditary or acquired pathological conditions. Hereditary angioneurotic edema is characterized by the absence of the C1 esterase inhibitor. This deficiency, besides being a genetic marker of the disease, plays a definite role in its pathogenesis. Inborn deficiencies of C2, C3, and C5 have been detected in apparently healthy individuals, and a decrease in C1q has been observed in patients with congenital agammaglobulinemia.

Acquired abnormalities of the complement system because of increased utilization are found in diseases such as systemic lupus erythematosus, acute and chronic glomerulonephritis, Goodpasture's syndrome, and autoimmune hemolytic anemia. Low complement levels have also been observed in the synovial fluid of some patients with rheumatoid arthritis who are seropositive for rheumatoid factor. Acquired abnormalities due to decreased synthesis of complement components have been detected in some patients with kidney or liver diseases, while low levels have also been observed in myasthenia gravis, renal allograft rejection, rheumatic fever, and paroxysmal nocturnal hemoglobinuria.

Whole-complement levels can be measured by the hemolytic assay, while complement components can be detected by several methods, such as immune hemolysis by the R reagent method or by the cellular intermediate method. Red cell antibody-complement reactions can be interrupted at various stages, obtaining cellular intermediate products that can be isolated and used to detect single complement components. Immunodiffusion in gel (immunoelectrophoresis or single radial immunodiffusion), and fluorescein- or ferritin-labeled antisera to individual components can also be used.

Although quantitation of complement components can be performed by some of these techniques, the most commonly employed methods in a clinical laboratory are single radial immunodiffusion and immune hemolysis using cellular intermediates. Since immunodiffusion methods detect the presence but not the activity of a complement protein, they should not be depended upon alone but must be integrated with the hemolytic assay.

Titration of Total Complement Activity in Human Serum

Standard Volume Method

Materials

1. Sheep erythrocytes sensitized with a 1:2000 dilution of rabbit antibody against sheep red cell stroma (EA), 5×10^8 cells per milliliter in TEAE buffer (p. 209)
2. Human serum. For determination of total hemolytic complement activity, 5-10 ml of clotted blood should be delivered to the laboratory immediately after being drawn. The blood is allowed to stand at room temperature for one hour and then refrigerated for one hour before centrifugation and separation of the serum. The test itself is set up and performed in an ice bath except during standard incubation and reading periods.
3. Triethanolamine (TEAE) buffer (p. 209)

4.   30-ml test tubes
5.   Pipettes, 1 ml and 5 ml

Method

1.   Prepare a 1:150 dilution of the human serum using TEAE buffer as diluent.
2.   Transfer 1.5-, 2.0-, 2.5-, 3.0-, 3.5-, and 4.0-ml portions of this dilution into a series of reaction test tubes.
3.   Add the required amount of TEAE buffer to bring the volume in each tube to 6.5 ml.
4.   Add exactly 1.0 ml of EA suspension (5×10^8 cells per milliliter) to all tubes. Final total volume in each reaction mixture will be 7.5 ml.
5.   Set up cell blank control by adding 1.0 ml of EA to 6.5 ml of buffer. Set up complete lysis control by adding 1.0 ml of EA to 6.5 ml distilled water.
6.   Incubate all reaction mixture tubes and controls at 37°C for one hour. Be sure to mix the contents in each tube frequently during the incubation period so that the cells will not be allowed to settle.
7.   After the incubation period, centrifuge the tubes at 600g for 10 minutes. Carefully pour off the supernatant fluid into appropriately labeled tubes. Read the hemoglobin color in the supernatant fluids photometrically at 415 mμ. Correct the readings for each reaction mixture and complete lysis control by subtracting cell blank readings. Determine the degree of lysis (y) for each tube by dividing the corrected optical density values by the corrected complete lysis value (y is the ratio of the optical density of lysed to unlysed cell supernatants so that $y = 1.0$ is complete lysis and $y = 0.5$ is 50% lysis).
8.   Using log-log graph paper, plot the value of $y/(1-y)$ for each reaction mixture against the corresponding amount of complement. Fit the best line to the experimental points and read the 50% lytic dose from the graph.
9.   The content of the complement is the number of 50% lytic doses (CH_{50} units) contained in 1 ml of the undiluted serum.

Small Volume Method. The reactions are carried out in a smaller volume, that is, 2.5 ml. It is commonly used for titration of guinea pig serum in connection with the complement fixation test but may also be used for measurement of complement levels in human serum, with some loss of precision as compared to the macromethod.

Materials

1.   EA suspension in TEAE buffer, 1×10^8 cells per milliliter

2. Human serum
3. Triethanolamine (TEAE) buffer (p. 209)
4. 10-ml test tubes
5. Pipettes, 1 ml

Method

1. Prepare a series of dilutions of the human serum to include 1:200, 1:250, 1:300, 1:400, 1:500, 1:600, and 1:800.
2. Transfer 2.0 ml of each dilution into separate labeled test tubes.
3. Add to each tube, 0.5 ml of EA suspension (1 x 10^8 cells per milliliter).
4. Set up a cell blank control by adding 0.5 ml of EA to 2 ml of buffer.
5. Set up a complete lysis control by adding 0.5 ml of EA to 2 ml of distilled water.
6. Incubate all reaction mixtures and controls at 37°C for 60 minutes. Be sure to mix the contents of each tube frequently during the incubation period so that the cells will not be allowed to settle.
7. After the incubation period add 5.0 ml of cold saline to each tube. Centrifuge at 2000 rpm for 10 minutes.
8. Carefully pour off the supernatant fluid into appropriately labeled tubes.
9. Read the hemoglobin color of the supernatant fluid photochemically at 415 mμ.
10. Correct the readings for each reaction mixture and complete lysis control by subtracting cell blank reading. Determine the degree of lysis for each tube by dividing the corrected optical density values by the corrected complete lysis value.
11. Using log-log graph paper, plot the values of $y/(1-y)$ for each reaction mixture against the corresponding concentration of complement. Fit the best line and read the 50% lytic dose.
12. The content of the complement is expressed as the number of 50% lytic doses (CH_{50} units) contained in 1 ml of the undiluted serum.

Measurement of Complement Components in Human Serum

Single Radial Immunodiffusion for C3 ($\beta_1 C$)

Materials

1. Immunodiffusion plates containing 1% agarose with goat antiserum against C3 ($\beta_1 C$) (Plates are prepared and wells are punched as described on p. 6)
2. Standard human serum containing a known amount of C3

3. Patient's serum
4. Microliter pipettes

Method

1. Prepare doubling serial dilutions of the standard and of the patient's serum in saline solution.
2. Fill three wells with separate dilutions of standard serum.
3. Fill three other wells with dilutions of patient's serum.
4. Cover plates and incubate at 37°C or room temperature in humidified chamber for 24 hours, then read diameters to the nearest 0.1 mm. On semi-log graph paper, plot the concentration in milligrams percent of C3 (β_1 C) on the logarithmic scale against the diameter of the standard on the arithmetic scale. Draw a curve to fit the observed points. From the standard curve, read off the diameter of the unknown sample and determine the amount of C3 (β_1 C) protein.

Hemolytic C4 Assay

Materials

1. Patient's serum
2. Normal human serum standard (NHS) (A standard containing known hemolytic activity of C4 should be used; this may be purified C4 component or a pool of normal human serum.)
3. C2 component (Cordis; diluted 1:10 in Gl-GVB 2+ buffer)
4. Whole complement (diluted 1:12.5 in EDTA-GVB buffer)
5. EAC1 guinea pig cells (1×10^8 cells per milliliter; Cordis)
6. G1-GVB 2+ buffer (p. 199)
7. EDTA-GVB buffer (p. 206)
8. Sterile distilled water
9. Microtiter plates
10. Pipettes and diluters (0.025 ml)
11. Plate shaker

Method

1. Using a marking pen, label a microtiter plate for the appropriate serial dilutions of the patient's serum and the normal human serum control. Allow 12 wells for each specimen per row. Also circle one well to be used for a 100% lysis control and one well to be used for a reagent lysis control. This will give two rows of 12 wells each and 2 miscellaneous wells.

2. Using a micropipette place one drop of Gl-GVB 2+ into all wells except the first well of each row and the 100% lysis control well. (Instructions for the 100% lysis control are under "9" below.) The reagent lysis well should receive two drops of the buffer.

3. Using separate pipettes place two drops of each sample to be tested (patient's serum and NHS) in the first well of each appropriate row. Prepare a serial twofold dilution by placing the diluters in the first wells and picking up a drop of the appropriate specimen. Place the diluters in the second well of the row, rotate to mix the sample, and lift to transfer to the next well. Repeat this procedure until the wells for each row are mixed.

Note: *The reagent lysis well receives no patient's serum or NHS at this point; however, all other reagents that will be added to the two specimen rows should also be added to the reagent lysis well.*

4. Add one drop of EAC1 guinea pig cells. Place the plate on a shaker at a moderate speed for 20 minutes at 30°C.

5. Add one drop of C2 component. Again mix on the plate shaker at 30°C for 10 minutes.

6. Add one drop of EDTA-GVB; then add one drop of diluted whole complement. Place the plate on the shaker for 60 minutes at 37°C.

7. Spin the plate in the special head of a refrigerated centrifuge at 1000 rpm for five minutes.

8. Determine the degree of lysis in each well by observing the size of the sedimented unlysed red cells and the color of the supernatant. C4 hemolysis titer is equal to the reciprocal of the highest dilution showing 50% (2+) lysis. The reagent lysis well should be negative.

9. Instructions for 100% lysis well: add one drop (0.025 ml) of EAC1 guinea pig cells, and four drops (0.025 ml = 1 drop) of sterile distilled water to this well.

REFERENCES

1. Kabat, E. A. and Mayer, M. M. *Experimental Immunochemistry* (Thomas: Springfield, Ill., 1961).

2. Nelson, R. A., Jensen, J., Gigli, I., and Tamura, N. Methods for the separation purification and measurement of nine components of hemolytic complement in guinea pig serum. *Immunochem. 3*, 111 (1966).

3. Schur, P. H. and Austen, K. F. Complement in human disease. *Ann. Rev. Med. 19*, 1 (1968).

Chapter 3

AGGLUTINATION REACTIONS

N. Rose   K. Wicher
P. Bigazzi   E. Gorzynski
W. Bartholomew   C. Abeyounis

Agglutination reactions are caused by the clumping of particulate antigens coated by their antibodies in the presence of certain electrolytes. Bacterial agglutination procedures are widely used in diagnostic bacteriology (Widal test for typhoid fever, Weil-Felix test for rickettsial infections, Wright test for brucellosis, etc.) and erythrocyte agglutination methods are employed for blood grouping (p. 71).

Methods for attaching soluble antigens to particles have been devised so that antibodies against these antigens can be demonstrated by the agglutination of the "sensitized" particles. A variety of "passive" agglutination techniques are currently used to detect antibodies to several antigens (γ globulins, DNA and other polynucleotides, thyroglobulin, growth hormone, TSH, gonadotropins, HAA, tuberculoprotein, etc.).

The mixed agglutination technique is based on the agglutination of two cell types (one, usually erythrocytes, functioning as an indicator) by an antibody directed to an antigen present on both types of cells. The introduction of an indicator system with antiglobulin reagents has made the test applicable to the detection of cell surface antigens and their corresponding antibodies.

Typically, agglutination procedures are characterized by great sensitivity.

ENTEROBACTERIAL AGGLUTINATION TEST

The etiologic diagnosis of an enterobacterial infection and of brucellosis and rickettsiosis is made best by isolating the pathogen from a suitable specimen and confirming the identity of this microorganism by employing biochemical and serological procedures. Frequently, isolation of the pathogen is impossible or impractical. In the latter situation, an etiologic diagnosis may be assisted by

45

identifying the presence and titer of antibodies in samples of the subject's serum. To this end, it is important that a serum specimen be obtained from the patient very early in the disease and be titrated against standardized bacterial antigens in parallel with serum sample(s) obtained later in the disease. An elevated titer of bacterial agglutinins may reflect a secondary, anamnestic or memory response that frequently accompanies a febrile episode or may reveal the etiologic agent of the infectious process involved. A single serum sample, in the absence of a careful assessment of the patient's history of immunization and infection, will yield limited or misleading information regarding the reason for the level of antibodies detected; the presence of antibodies may indicate a current or previous infection or a history of immunization against the pathogen in question; a rise in antibody during the course of an infection may be meaningful.

Two quantitative procedures are currently employed in detecting the level of antibodies to enterobacteria, brucella, and rickettsia: the slide agglutination test and the tube agglutination test. These tests are based on the principle that bacteria will aggregate in the presence of antibodies to their antigenic determinants; standardized bacterial antigens are employed as indicator.

Materials

1. Standardized bacterial antigens (commercially available):
    A. *Brucella abortus* antigens
    B. Proteus OX19, OX2, and OXK antigens (2)
    C. Salmonella group A (O antigens 1, 2, 12)
    D. Salmonella group B (O antigens 4, 5, 12)
    E. Salmonella groups C and C2 (O antigens 6, 7, 8, Vi)
    F. Salmonella group D (O antigens 1, 9, 12, Vi)
    G. Salmonella groups E1-E4 (O antigens 1, 3, 15, 19, 34)
    H. Paratyphoid A antigen (flagellar a)
    I. Paratyphoid B antigen (flagellar b, 1, 2)
    J. Paratyphoid C antigen (flagellar c, 1, 5)
    K. Typhoid H antigen (flagellar d)
2. Physiological saline solution, pH 7.2
3. Waterbaths maintained at 37°C and 50°C
4. Glass slides (9 x 14 in.)
5. Test tubes ca. 10 x 100 mm and 20 x 100 mm; test-tube (agglutinating) racks
6. Pipettes (0.2, 1, 2, 5, and 10 ml)

Method

1. Slide agglutination test:
    A. Using a 0.2-ml pipette, deliver 0.08, 0.04, 0.02, 0.01, and 0.005 ml
        patient's serum to 30-mm squares or rings marked on the 9 x 14 in.
        glass slide. Repeat this on as many slides as there are antigens to be
        used.
    B. Shake the vials of standardized bacterial antigens to mix thoroughly
        the contents. The dropper provided with each antigen has been stan-
        dardized to deliver approximately 0.03 ml; place one drop on each
        volume of serum in each row.
    C. With individual applicator sticks or toothpicks for each marked area
        containing serum dilution and antigen, mix the contents. This quan-
        tity of antigen (0.03 ml), when mixed with the varying quantities of
        serum, will give dilutions approximating those obtained in the test-
        tube method, that is, 1:20, 1:40, 1:80, 1:160, and 1:320. Further
        dilutions may be prepared by employing a 1:10 dilution of serum in
        saline and utilizing the identical volumes of serum shown in A. In this
        latter procedure, the first dilution will be equivalent to 1:200.
    D. Rotate the slide over a lighted surface (which provides heat and
        maximum visibility) for three to four minutes and, concurrently,
        observe for agglutination.
    E. The smallest quantity (highest dilution) of serum agglutinating more
        than 50% of the standardized bacterial antigen is considered the end
        point or titer.
    F. Interpretation of the test results will be considered below.
2. Tube agglutination test: since the sera usually are tested with several
    antigens, a parallel dilution method is utilized. The procedure shown below
    allows for testing aliquot serum dilutions with nine standardized bacterial
    antigens; larger volumes of this master dilution system will be required if
    more than nine antigens are to be employed.
    A. Preparations of master dilutions
        (1) Set up nine 20 x 100 mm test tubes in a rack; number them from
             1 to 9.
        (2) Add 8 ml of saline to tube 1 and 5 ml to tubes 2-9.
        (3) Mix 2 ml of undiluted patient's serum with the saline in tube 1;
             transfer 4 ml of this mixture to tube 2 and mix. Continue to
             transfer and mix 5-ml volumes to the remaining tubes. Note that
             the total volume of serum dilution in tubes 1-8 is 5.0 ml and in
             tube 9, 10 ml. It is obvious that if further dilutions of serum are
             required to establish an end point or titer, tube 10 may serve as

the starting dilution.

B.   Procedure for parallel agglutination tests

(1) Set up nine 10 x 100 mm test tubes in each of 10 rows in test-tube racks; number the first row A1-A10, the second row B1-B10, the third row C1-C10 and so on; the ninth row will be numbered I1-I10. Each lettered row will represent a different antigen series.

(2) Add 0.5 ml of saline to tube 10 in each lettered row.

(3) With a 5-ml pipette, transfer 0.5 ml of the highest dilution (tube 9 of the master-dilution series, A3 above) to each tube numbered 9 in the lettered series (B1 above). With the same pipette, transfer 0.5 ml of the next, lower dilution to each tube numbered 8 in the lettered series. By starting with the highest dilution and working backward, the same pipette may be employed throughout the procedure with little concern for carrying over any appreciable amount of antibody.

(4) Dilute each selected standardized bacterial antigen 1:100 with physiological saline; shake each antigen vial thoroughly before withdrawing a quantity for dilution. Add 0.5 ml of diluted antigen to all tubes. Since the antigens used in agglutination tests are subject to variations, it is necessary that control tests, using positive antisera of known titer, be carried out occasionally as a check on the agglutinability of the test antigens.

(5) Shake the rack of tubes to mix antigen and serum thoroughly. The final serum dilutions now range as follows:

Tube	Final serum dilution
1	1:10
2	1:20
3	1:40
4	1:80
5	1:160
6	1:320
7	1:640
8	1:1280
9	1:2560
10	control

Place the racks in a waterbath at the temperatures and the time periods indicated below:

Antigen	Time and temperature
Salmonella H	2 hr., 50°C
Salmonella O	18-24 hr., 50°C
Proteus	2hr., 37°C, then 12-16 hr., 4°C
Brucella	24 hr., 37°C

C. Reading agglutination tests
   (1) Remove racks from the waterbath or refrigerator; do not disturb settled antigen.
   (2) Observe every tube for clearing of the supernatant fluid and the amount and character of the sedimented and agglutinated particles. This is accomplished best by holding the tubes over a concave mirror, observing the magnified reflection, and examining the following three tubes concurrently: Patient's serum dilution, negative (saline) control (tube 10), and positive serum control.
   (3) While these three tubes are held over the mirror, they should be shaken gently; H agglutinins produce large floccular aggregates that are broken up easily; O agglutinins produce granular or small flaky aggregates that are not easily broken up.
   (4) Recording results: Complete agglutination with complete clearing of the supernatant fluid indicates that all of the bacteria have agglutinated: this is a 4+ reaction. Decreasing amounts of agglutination and increasing cloudiness of the supernatant fluid are recorded as 3+, 2+, and 1+ reactions. In a negative reaction, there is no evidence of agglutination; that is, in the tube the same density as in the saline-antigen control tube is observed.
   (5) Determination of titer: The titer of the serum is designated as the highest dilution of serum (the smallest quantity of undiluted serum) that exhibits a 50% degree of agglutination (a 2+ reaction). Table 3.1 gives several examples of test evaluations.
3. Interpretation of results: It is not practical to assign positive or negative values to arbitrary titers in any agglutination test, since many factors--for example, a history of infection or active immunization, the day after infection when the specimen was taken, the presence of natural agglutinins--may cause variable results. Therefore, only a rise in titer over a period

Table 3.1.   Sample Agglutination Reactions

Serum Dilution	Serum 1	Serum 2	Serum 3
1:20	4+	3+	4+
1:40	3+	2+	3+c
1:80	2+	2+b	1+
1:160	2+a	1+	1+
1:320	--	1+	--
1:640	--	--	--
Saline	--	--	--

a titer 160.
b titer 80.
c titer 40.

of time (during the course of an infection) is usually significant. Interpretation of positive results will vary with the disease involved. The following guide may be helpful:
A. Typhoid fever: O antibodies disappear in approximately one year in actively immunized individuals; therefore, a titer of 50 or more indicates recent immunization or current infection, while an increase (fourfold or more) during the course of infection supports the likelihood of a current infection. H antibodies persist in vaccinated subjects and are not elevated during current infection; therefore, a titer of 80 or more with H antigen only indicates past infection, active immunization, or an anamnestic reaction.
B. Brucellosis: A titer of 160 or more usually suggests infection, past or present.
C. Rickettsiosis: For the serological diagnosis of rickettsial infections, antigens from specific strains of *Proteus* are employed. A titer of 320 with OX19 suggests a typhus fever, and a titer of 320 with OX2 suggests Rocky Mountain spotted fever; a rising titer is conclusive evidence. Agglutination with *Proteus* OXK may be diagnostic for tsutsugamushi fever but may also indicate relapsing fever.

REFERENCES

1. Bailey, W. R. and Scott, E. G. *Diagnostic Microbiology*, (3rd ed.) (Mosby: St. Louis, Mo., 1970).
2. Davis, B. D., Dulbecco, R., Eisen, H. N., Ginsberg, H. S., and Wood, W. B., Jr. *Microbiology* (Harper and Row: New York, 1967).

INDIRECT (PASSIVE) AGGLUTINATION

Soluble antigens can be used in an agglutination reaction when attached to an inert carrier (passive agglutination). Erythrocytes have been found to be among the most convenient carriers. Red blood cells sensitized with specific antibodies are used to detect antibodies to γ globulins (Waaler-Rose and Wasser-Vaughan tests for rheumatoid factor). Untreated red blood cells can adsorb certain soluble antigens, such as penicillin (penicillin hemagglutination test) or bacterial polysaccharide (bacterial hemagglutination test). For adsorption of soluble protein antigens, however, the surface of the erythrocyte has to be modified; basically this can be accomplished in two ways. In the first method, tannic acid is used to alter the red blood cell's surface and enable it to adsorb protein antigens (tanned-cell hemagglutination test). In the other method, the antigens are coupled to the erythrocyte surface by chemical linkage, using chromic chloride, difluorodinitrobenzine, or bis-diazotized benzidine (bis-diazotized benzidine hemagglutination test).

Latex and bentonite particles can also be used as carriers for soluble antigens (latex agglutination test, bentonite agglutination test).

Tanned-Cell Hemagglutination Test for Thyroid Antibodies

For the assay of small quantities of antibody, the tanned-cell hemagglutination test provides an extremely sensitive technique. Tannic acid acts on erythrocytes in such a way as to cause them to take up protein antigens. Once tannic-acid-treated erythrocytes are mixed with the proper concentration of antigen, they acquire a protein "overcoat." Washed, coated erythrocytes can then be added to serial dilutions of a patient's serum in order to measure the titer of antibody.

In a modification of the method, the process of titration (microtitration) is accomplished using minute quantities of reagents. Transparent plastic plates containing small, specially-shaped cups are used instead of racks of test tubes. Specially constructed and calibrated "loops" capable of picking up constant volumes of fluid and making dilutions are used instead of the standard pipette.

Special pipette droppers are calibrated to deliver an accurate volume of fluid to the cups.

Macromethod

Materials

1. Human group O erythrocytes (HRBC). Collect 10 ml of human blood in 2.0 ml of standard ACD solution. The HRBC may be used from three days to two weeks after collection.
2. Phosphate-buffered saline solution (PBS), pH 7.2 (p. 205)
3. Tannic acid solution in PBS (p. 208)
4. Normal rabbit serum (NRS) diluent. Inactivate pooled normal rabbit serum for 30 minutes at 56°C and dilute 1:100 in PBS.
5. Pooled human-thyroid crude extract (p. 209)
6. Patient's serum and control sera (inactivated 30 minutes at 56°C)
7. Test tubes (12 x 75 mm and 16 x 150 mm)
8. Centrifuge tubes, graduated, 15 ml
9. Pipettes, 1 ml, 5 ml, and 10 ml

Method

1. Wash HRBC three times by sedimenting the cells in the centrifuge at 1500 rpm (800 g) for five minutes, using the horizontal head of a table top clinical centrifuge. After each centrifugation, remove the supernatant and resuspend in fresh saline. Transfer washed cells to 15-ml graduated centrifuge tube and pack by centrifugation at 1500 rpm in the clinical centrifuge. Prepare a 4% suspension in PBS.
2. Combine 5 ml of 4% HRBC suspension with 5 ml of 1:25,000 tannic acid. Mix by inversion, and allow to stand at room temperature for 30 minutes. On the side of the tube, mark the level of the fluid. Wash three times, using gentle centrifugation.

Note: *Washing should be carried out in PBS. Keep erythrocytes from any contact with protein such as NRS diluent. Also, take care to resuspend cells gently but completely between each washing.*

3. Add 0.1 ml of human-thyroid crude extract to 5.0 ml of PBS in a 50-ml test tube, and place in boiling water bath for exactly two minutes. After boiling, cool tube under running water and add 15.0 ml cold PBS.
4. After third washing of tanned cells, discard supernatant and add PBS to

mark, giving 10 ml of a 2% suspension. Mix by inversion, and add 5.0 ml of tanned cells and 5.0 ml of 1:200 dilution of thyroid extract in a 16 x 100 mm test tube. Boyden's original recommendation called for coating at pH 6.4. While this pH is optimal for certain antigens, thyroglobulin seems to attach more efficiently at pH 7.2. The proper concentration of antigen for coating must be determined by trial and error for each batch of antigen. In the above test, purified thyroglobulin may be substituted for crude thyroid extract. Prepare one tube of "uncoated cells" by combining 5 ml of tanned cells with 5 ml NRS diluent. Mark fluid level of both tubes and restore to this level after washing. Allow coated cells (and "uncoated" control cells) to stand at room temperature for 30 minutes. Wash three times in NRS diluent, and after washing, bring to volume with NRS, providing 10 ml of a 1% cell suspension.

5.   Prepare two rows of ten 12 x 75 mm test tubes. Prepare serial doubling dilutions (volume 0.1 ml) of the antiserum in NRS diluent, starting with a dilution of 1:10. The last tube on each row should receive 0.1 ml of NRS diluent only. Add 0.1 ml of tanned, coated HRBC to the first row of ten tubes. Add 0.1 ml of uncoated HRBC to the second row. Shake well and incubate at room temperature for 3 hours.

Protocol 3.1.   Tanned Cell Hemagglutination, Macromethod

| | Antiserum | Tanned HRBC | |
Tube	Dilution (0.1 ml)	Thyroid-coated (0.1 ml)	Uncoated (0.1 ml)
1	1:10		
2	1:20		
3	1:40		
4	1:80		
5	1:160		
6	1:320		
7	1:640		
8	1:1280		
9	1:2560		
10	control		

6. After 3 hours, read the tubes by observing the pattern of sedimentation on the bottom of the tube (Fig. 3.1). After the first reading has been taken, transfer the tubes to a refrigerator for overnight incubation at 4°C. A second reading is taken in the morning, after which the tubes are shaken and re-read after 3 hours of further incubation at room temperature.

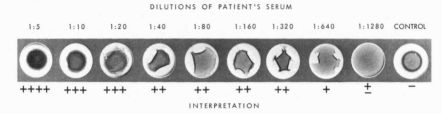

DILUTIONS OF PATIENT'S SERUM

1:5   1:10   1:20   1:40   1:80   1:160   1:320   1:640   1:1280   CONTROL

++++   +++   +++   ++   ++   ++   ++   +   ±   —

INTERPRETATION

Fig. 3.1.

Micromethod

Materials

1. Plates, microtiter–conical bottom or "U" plates (Cooke Engineering Company)
2. 0.025-ml diluters, standardized prior to using in test
3. 0.025-ml droppers
4. For other materials, see Macromethod (p. 52)

Method

1. Tanning and coating of erythrocytes are carried out as for the tube test, except that the final concentration of the erythrocyte suspension is 2%.
2. Prepare a 1:5 dilution of patient's serum in a test tube, using NRS diluent.
3. 0.025 ml of NRS diluent is placed in wells 1-12.
4. Using a diluter, take a loopful of 1:5 patient's serum dilution, and place it in the first well. Twirl diluter 8 times, carefully remove from well and transfer to next well again mixing 8 times. Continue in this manner through the first 9 wells.
5. Place 0.025 ml of the 1:5 patient's serum dilution in well 11. Mix as in previous step and then transfer a loopful into well 12. These two wells are controls using tanned uncoated erythrocytes.
6. Add 0.025 ml tanned, coated erythrocytes to wells 1-10. Add 0.025 ml tanned, uncoated erythrocytes to wells 11 and 12.

Protocol 3.2.   Tanned Cell Hemagglutination, Micromethod

Well	Antiserum dilution	Erythrocytes
1	1:10	
2	1:20	
3	1:40	
4	1:80	
5	1:160	Tanned
6	1:320	and coated
7	1:640	
8	1:1280	
9	1:2560	
10	0	
11	1:10	Tanned only
12	1:20	

7. Tap plate gently to mix.
8. Cover plate with plastic, punching hole over each well with hypodermic needle to avoid condensation.
9. Incubate plates at room temperature until patterns settle (usually one hour is sufficient), then overnight at 4°C.
10. Read the pattern of sedimentation as for the tube test.

REFERENCES

1. Boyden, S. The absorption of proteins on erythrocytes treated with tannic acid and the subsequent hemagglutination by anti-protein sera. *J. Exp. Med. 93*, 107 (1951).
2. Haber, J. A. and Rose, N. R. Comparative studies of indirect hemagglutination. *Int. Arch. Aller. Appl. Immunol. 34*, 303 (1968).
3. Stavitsky, A. B. Micromethods for the study of proteins and antibodies. I. Procedure and general applications of hemagglutination and hemagglutination-inhibition reactions with tannic acid and protein-treated red blood

cells. *J. Immunol. 72*, 360 (1954).

4.   Takátsy, G. The use of spiral loops in serological and virological micro-
      methods. *Acta Microbiol. Acad. Sci. Hung. 3*, 191 (1955).
5.   Witebsky, E. and Rose, N. R. Studies on organ specificity. IV. Production
      of rabbit thyroid antibodies in the rabbit. *J. Immunol. 76*, 408 (1956).

Bis-Diazotized Benzidine Hemagglutination Test

Materials

1.   Rabbit RBC, collected in Alsever's solution
2.   Bis-diazotized benzidine (BDB) solution (p. 197)
3.   Phosphate-buffered saline solution (PBS) pH 7.2
4.   Normal rabbit serum (NRS) diluent (normal rabbit serum inactivated and
      diluted 1:100 in PBS)
5.   Antigen
6.   Antiserum and control sera
7.   Phosphate buffer 0.15M, pH 7.3 (p. 205)
8.   Test tubes, 12 x 75 mm and 10 x 150 mm
9.   Pipettes, 1 ml, 5 ml, 10 ml

Method

1.   Wash rabbit RBC three times in physiological saline solution, and make a
      50% suspension of the RBC in normal saline. Mix 0.1 ml of the 50%
      suspension with 0.5 ml BDB diluted in phosphate buffer. The dilution
      factor of the BDB must be determined empirically using a known antigen-
      antibody system.
2.   To the RBC-BDB mixture, add 3 ml of the proper dilution of the antigen
      solution diluted in phosphate buffer. The antigen concentration must also
      be determined empirically.
3.   Prepare the control suspension of RBC using 3 ml of buffer, 0.1 ml of 50%
      RBC, and 0.5 ml of diluent.
4.   Incubate both the coated and the uncoated RBC (control) for 15 minutes
      at room temperature and centrifuge them for 5 minutes at 800 g. Remove
      the supernatant, wash the RBC once with an excess of diluent, and then
      resuspend the RBC in 2.5 ml of diluent.
5.   Prepare two rows of ten 12 x 75 mm tubes. Prepare serial twofold dilutions
      (volume 0.5 ml) of the antisera in the diluent starting with a dilution of
      1:10. Tube 10 is a control of the coated RBC and will contain only 0.5 ml

of diluent. Proceed in the same way with control 2.

6. Add 0.05 ml of the coated RBC suspension to each tube in row 1, including the control tube. Add 0.05 ml of the uncoated RBC suspension to each tube in row 2. Shake the tubes and incubate them at room temperature for two hours.

Protocol 3.3.   Bis-Diazotized Benzidine Hemagglutination Test

Tube	Antiserum Dilution	BDB-Treated RBC Coated	Uncoated
1	1:10		
2	1:20		
3	1:40		
4	1:80		
5	1:160		
6	1:320		
7	1:640		
8	1:1280		
9	1:2560		
10	control		

7. Read the test for passive agglutination as in the tanned-cell hemagglutination test. Place the tubes in the refrigerator overnight and take a second reading in the morning.

REFERENCES

1. Brinckerhoff, C. E. and Rose, N. R. Detection of rabbit pancreas-specific iso-antibodies by bis-diazotized benzidine hemagglutination. *J. Immunol.* *102*, 1208 (1969).
2. Butler, W. T. Hemagglutination studies with formalinized erythrocytes. Effect of bis-diazo-benzidine and tannic acid treatment on sensitization by soluble antigen. *J. Immunol. 90*, 663 (1963).
3. Gordon, J., Rose, B., and Sehon, A. H. Detection of non-precipitating

antibodies in sera of individuals allergic to ragweed pollen by an in vitro method. *J. Exptl. Med. 108*, 37 (1958).
4.   Haber, J. A. and Rose, N. R. Comparative studies of indirect hemagglutination. *Int. Arch. Aller. & Appl. Immunol. 34*, 303 (1968).
5.   Pressman, D., Campbell, D. H., and Pauling, L. The agglutination of intact azoerythrocytes by antisera homologous to the attached groups. *J. Immunol. 44*, 101 (1942).
6.   Stavitsky, A. B. and Arquilla, E. R. Procedure and applications of hemagglutination inhibition reactions with bis-diazotized benzidine and protein conjugated red blood cells. *J. Immunol. 74*, 306 (1955).

Hemagglutination Procedures for HAA and HA Antibody

Double-diffusion procedures for HAA and for antibody to HAA (HA antibody) are time consuming and not very sensitive. Counterimmunoelectrophoresis (p. 19) gives results within two hours and is five times more sensitive. Complement fixation also gives results within two hours but is 100 times more sensitive for HAA and 20 times more sensitive for the antibody. Radioimmunoassay procedures seem to be as sensitive but are more time consuming and require special equipment and reagents.

Recently Vyas and Shulman (1) have introduced a hemagglutination technique. This procedure is based on the use of erythrocytes coated with HAA (coupled by chromic chloride to the red cells) to detect the antibody to this antigen. The method is 2000 times more sensitive than double diffusion, 100 times more sensitive than complement fixation, and requires only small amounts of serum and antigen-coated cells (2).

The demonstration of HAA in the serum of patients is based on the inhibition of the agglutination of HAA-coated cells and a standard antiserum to HAA. The combination of a known, small amount (0.025 ml) of standard hyperimmune anti-HAA with a test serum before the addition of HAA-coated erythrocytes will neutralize anti-HAA and prevent agglutination of the coated erythrocytes if HAA is present in the test serum. This method is more sensitive than double diffusion and as sensitive as complement fixation.

Hemagglutination Assay for HA Antibody

Materials

1.   HAA-coated red blood cells, human O Rh-negative (Virge reagents) and control red blood cells

2. TAP buffer (Tween 80, serum bovine albumin, PVP) (p. 208). This buffer promotes better red-cell settling patterns.
3. Patients' sera and control sera (known positive and negative)
4. V-shaped microtiter plates
5. 0.025-ml loops and diluters

Method

1. 0.025 ml of cells coated with HAA are added to 0.025 ml of serial twofold dilutions of patient's serum made in TAP buffer.
2. Incubate reactions one hour at room temperature.
3. Centrifuge microtiter plates at 1200 rpm for approximately 30 seconds. Smoothly accelerate to desired speed, turn off power, and allow centrifuge to slow without braking.
4. Keep microtiter plates on an angle of $60°$ for 15-20 minutes before reading. A discrete button of agglutinated cells will be seen as a dot, and a smooth line of cells that streamed down the vertex of the V-shaped well in a microtiter plate constitutes no agglutination. Cells that are completely agglutinated remain as a small dot in the bottom of the well or occasionally fall down as a clump.

Hemagglutination Inhibition Test for HAA

Materials

1. Same as in hemagglutination assay for HA antibody.

Method

1. The amount of antibody to be used in hemagglutination inhibition is four times the amount of the highest dilution completely agglutinating in the hemagglutination assay for HA antibody. Therefore, if the highest dilution that agglutinates erythrocytes is 1:16,000, then a 1:4000 dilution (4 units of antibody) of this serum is used as a standard antibody in the hemagglutination-inhibition test.
2. Dilute test sera 1:2, 1:10, 1:100, and 1:200 (these dilutions will vary). Make all preliminary dilutions in NaCl and the final dilution in TAP buffer.
3. Add 0.025 ml of serum dilutions and 0.025 ml of standard antibody dilution (4 units) in the wells of the plate. Include one known, positive control and one normal, human serum. Include standard hyperimmune anti-HAA serum in 4-, 2-, and 1-unit concentrations (1:4,000; 1:8,000; and

1:16,000 dilutions).

4. Allow plate to set for five minutes before adding HAA-coated erythrocytes (this time and sequence of addition of reagents is necessary to provide time for the combination of antibody with antigen, if the latter is present in the patient's serum).

5. The remainder of the test is carried out in the same manner as in the hemagglutination assay for HA antibody.

6. A reaction is considered "positive" when the cells are streaming down the side of the well, that is, when the presence of the HAA inhibits hemagglutination by the standard serum. A reaction is considered "negative" when the agglutinated cells remain as a button on the bottom of the well, that is, when there is no inhibition of agglutination. A titer of 4 or greater is considered positive for HAA.

REFERENCES

1. Vyas, G. N. and Schulman, N. R. Hemagglutination assay for antigen and antibody associated with viral hepatitis. *Science 170*, 332 (1970).

2. Wegmann, T. G. and Smithies, O. A simple hemagglutination system requiring small amounts of red cells and antibodies. *Transfusion 6*, 67 (1966).

Penicillin Hemagglutination Test

Over 35 cases of nephropathy due to penicillin, methicillin, and ampicillin have been reported. In the described cases, circulating antibodies to penicillin or derivatives were found. Therefore, a test for detecting such circulating antibodies in patients' sera is important in a diagnostic laboratory.

Materials

1. Patients' sera
2. Human O Rh negative red blood cells
3. Potassium penicillin G, USP 200,000 units (powder)
4. Sodium barbital buffer, pH 8.4 (p. 206)
5. Phosphate-buffered saline solution, pH 7.3 (PBS) (p. 205)
6. Normal rabbit serum (NRS) diluent. Absorb the NRS with O Rh negative red blood cells, thereafter inactivate at 56°C for 30 minutes. Prepare each time fresh diluent by diluting the absorbed inactivated NRS 1:100.
7. Test tubes, 12 x 75 mm
8. Pipettes, 1 ml

Method

1. The adsorption of penicillin to red blood cells is performed 24 hours prior to the test. Add 2.5 ml of packed erythrocytes to 200,000 units of penicillin, add 2.5 ml of sodium barbital buffer to the flask, and mix thoroughly. Incubate in 37°C waterbath for one hour; keep in refrigerator overnight.
2. Make serial dilutions of the serum to be tested in two rows using diluent. The starting dilution should be 1:2, and the volume, 0.3 ml. Include a positive and negative control.
3. Wash penicillin-coated cells three times in 0.15 M PBS. Prepare a 3% suspension of both coated and uncoated red blood cells to tubes of the first row and 0.1 ml of the uncoated red blood cells into tubes of the second row. Shake, incubate at room temperature for 15 minutes, then centrifuge at 1000 rpm for 3 minutes.
4. Read the agglutination reaction in each tube individually, shaking very gently. Evaluate the reactions in the same way as tanned-cell hemagglutination (p. 53).

REFERENCES

1. Baldwin, D. S., Levine, B. B., McCluskey, R. T., and Gallo, G. R. Renal failure and interstitial nephritis due to penicillin and methicillin. *N. E. J. Med.* 279, 1245 (1968).
2. Levine, B. B., Fellner, M. J., and Levytska, V. Benzylpenicilloyl-specific serum antibodies to penicillin in man. I. Development of sensitive hemagglutination assay method and haptenic specifications of antibodies. *J. Immunol.* 96, 707 (1966).
3. Levine, B. B., Fellner, M. J., Levytska, V., Franklin, E. C., and Alisberg, N. II. Sensitivity of hemagglutination assay method, molecular classes of antibodies detected and antibody titers of randomly selected patients. *J. Immunol.* 96, 719 (1966).
4. Wicher, K., Tannenberg, A., and Rose, N. R. Ampicillin nephropathy. *J. A. M. A.* 218, 449 (1971).

Bacterial Hemagglutination Test

Infectious diseases caused by species or serogroups of *Salmonella*, *Shigella*, and enteropathogenic *Escherichia coli* are encountered sporadically or in epidemic forms in most communities throughout the civilized world. Mild and subclinical infections often escape detection. The etiological diagnosis of these diseases is based on the isolation of the etiologic agent from a suitable specimen and the identification of this isolate by biochemical and serological procedures. To support the presence of an infectious process caused by a specific microorganism, serum specimens are assessed for antibodies early and during the course of the disease. The bacterial hemagglutination test (1) is a sensitive procedure for demonstrating enterobacterial antibodies (2-4). The method is based on the observation that erythrocytes readily absorb O antigens of *Enterobacteriaceae* and thus become agglutinable in the presence of the corresponding bacterial antibodies. This method is more sensitive than the conventional bacterial agglutination procedure. In addition, it is possible to modify erythrocytes with many antigens and thus have available a multivalent indicator for the demonstration or screening of antibody responses in subjects with clinical or subclinical enterobacterial infections. Moreover, enterobacterial antisera may be employed effectively in the hemagglutination test to supplement or confirm the identity of an isolated microorganism. Described below are the materials and methods employed in the bacterial hemagglutination test.

Materials

1. Antigens. Smooth strains of enteric bacteria are grown on brain veal agar in Kolle flasks for 18 hours at 37°C; growth in each flask is suspended in 25 ml of phosphate hemagglutination buffer, pH 7.3 (Difco). The suspensions are heated in boiling water for one hour and then centrifuged at 23,500 g (4°C) for 30 minutes; clear supernatant fluids are decanted and kept frozen until used.
2. Antisera obtained from patients or immunized rabbits
3. Indicator erythrocytes. Human erythrocytes (HRBC), group O Rh − are obtained (using sodium citrate or heparin as anticoagulant) from healthy subjects. One volume of this whole blood is washed three times with up to 20 volumes of phosphate hemagglutination buffer; the final concentration of HRBC is 2.5%.
4. Test tubes 12 x 75 mm
5. Pipettes, 1 ml

Method

1. To the washed sediment of HRBC, add 19.5 volumes of antigen. Incubate this mixture in a waterbath at 37°C for 30 minutes, wash three times with about 20 volumes of phosphate buffer, and resuspend the washed HRBC

sediment in 19.5 volumes of buffer. These resuspended erythrocytes possess adsorbed antigens and will be agglutinated in the presence of antibodies specific for the antigen employed in the treatment of erythrocytes, described above.

2. Mix serum (0.2 ml) in serial twofold dilutions with 0.2 ml of antigentreated erythrocytes in 12 x 100 mm test tubes. The mixtures are incubated in a waterbath at 37°C for 30 minutes and then centrifuged at 1300 g for 2 minutes. Each tube is shaken individually and gently, and the presence or absence of hemagglutination is compared with positive and negative control tubes. Clumping of 70-100% of the HRBC is recorded as ++++ agglutination; barely visible hemagglutination is assigned a + reading; and depending upon the extent of agglutination between the + and ++++ extremes, levels of ++ and +++ are established arbitrarily.

3. The O specificity of the hemagglutination observed is determined by the inhibition test. In this procedure, 0.2 ml of the O antigen in question is mixed with the serum dilutions. This mixture is incubated in a waterbath at 37°C for 30 minutes prior to the addition of antigen-treated erythrocytes; the absence or reduction of hemagglutination, in the presence of antigeninhibitor, and the observation of hemagglutination in the absence of antigen inhibitor reflects O specificity.

REFERENCES

1. Neter, E. Bacterial hemagglutination and hemolysis. *Bact. Rev. 20*, 166 (1956).

2. ——————. Indirect bacterial hemagglutination and its application to the study of bacterial antigens and serologic diagnosis. *Path. Microbiol. 28*, 859 (1965).

3. Neter, E., Harris, A. H., and Drislane, A. M. The detection of enterobacterial infection in institutionalized children by means of the hemagglutination test. *Am. J. Pub. Health 55*, 1164 (1965).

4. Kunin, C. M., Beard, M. V. and Halmagyi, N. E. Evidence for a common hapten associated with endotoxin fractions of *E. coli* and other *Enterobacteriaceae. Proc. Soc. Exptl. Biol. Med. 111*, 160 (1962).

Agglutination of Sensitized Sheep Erythrocytes (Waaler-Rose Test)

The serological diagnosis of rheumatoid arthritis (RA) is based on an observation reported by Waaler in 1939. He found that sera from patients suffering from RA contained a factor, subsequently called rheumatoid factor (RF), capable of agglutinating sheep erythrocytes sensitized by a rabbit anti-sheep erythrocyte serum. This phenomenon was rediscovered by Rose and his associates, and they applied it to the diagnosis of RA. Later it was found that RF could react not only with γ globulin of rabbit origin, but also with γ globulin from other species including man. This led Waller and Vaughan to develop another hemagglutination test for the detection of RF. This test utilizes human Rh+ erythrocytes sensitized by human incomplete Rh antibodies.

RA serology was further advanced by Heller and his associates who introduced the principle of passive hemagglutination for the detection of RF. In this procedure, erythrocytes treated with tannic acid are coated with γ globulin. Singer and Plotz extended the use of passive hemagglutination by employing inert particles as a carrier of the antigen. In their procedure, latex particles are coated with γ globuin.

Materials

1. RA serum and normal human serum
2. 2% suspension of sheep red blood cells (SRBC)
3. Rabbit anti-SRBC serum (amboceptor) appropriately diluted. The SRBC are sensitized by a subagglutinating dose of anti-SRBC serum. The proper dilution is determined in a preliminary test in which various dilutions of the anti-SRBC serum are tested against SRBC.
4. 0.15 M saline solution

Method

1. In a 16 x 100 mm test tube, mix 3 ml of 2% SRBC with 3 ml of the appropriate (e.g. 1:4000) dilution of the anti-SRBC serum (sensitized SRBC). In another tube, mix 3 ml of 2% SRBC with 3 ml of saline (unsensitized SRBC). Incubate the two tubes in a waterbath at $37°C$ for 15 minutes.
2. For each serum to be tested, set up two rows with 12 tubes in each row. Label the tubes in the first row a_1 through a_{12}, and label the tubes in the second row b_1 through b_{12}. Place 0.9 ml of saline in tube a_1 and 0.4 ml saline in tubes a_2-a_{11}. Place 0.2 ml saline in tubes a_{12} and b_{12}, these are the control tubes for the sensitized and unsensitized SRBC, respectively.
3. Place 0.1 ml of the serum to be tested in tube a_1 and mix thoroughly to obtain a 1:10 dilution. Remove 0.8 ml from tube a_1. Place 0.2 ml in tube b_1, 0.4 ml in tube a_2, and discard the remaining 0.2 ml. Mix thoroughly the contents of tube a_2. Remove 0.6 ml from tube a_2, and place 0.2 ml in tube

b_2 and 0.4 ml in tube a_3. Mix thoroughly the contents of tube a_3. Repeat last step through tube a_{11}. Remove 0.6 ml from tube a_{11}, place 0.2 ml in tube b_{11}, and discard the rest.

4. Add 0.2 ml of sensitized SRBC (from step 1) to all tubes of row A. Add 0.2 ml of unsensitized SRBC (from step 1) to all tubes of row B. Shake well the rack containing the tubes and incubate overnight at $4°C$.

5. Bring the tubes to room temperature, and after 30 minutes read for agglutination of SRBC after gently shaking the tubes. The degree of agglutination is graded from 1+ to 4+.

Latex Agglutination

Tube Test

Materials

1. Suspension of latex particles (0.81 μ)
2. Borate buffer, pH 8.2 (RA-Test, Hyland)
3. 1% Fraction II (FII) of pooled human plasma in borate buffer
4. RA serum and normal human serum
5. Test tubes, 12 x 75 mm
6. Pipettes, 1 ml

Method

1. To 20 ml of 1% of FII, add 0.2 ml of the suspension of latex particles. Allow the mixture to stand at room temperature for 10 minutes.
2. Prepare a 1:10 dilution of each serum to be tested by mixing in a tube 0.9 ml of buffer and 0.1 ml of serum.
3. For each serum, place 10 tubes in a rack and label them 1 through 10. Add 0.2 ml of buffer to all tubes. Add 0.2 ml of serum dilution to tube 1 and mix thoroughly. Transfer 0.2 ml from tube 1 to tube 2, and mix thoroughly. Repeat last step through tube 9. Remove 0.2 ml from tube 9 and discard. (Tubes 1-9 contain 0.2 ml of serum at dilutions from 1:20 to 1:5120; tube 10, the antigen control, contains only 0.2 ml of buffer.)
4. To each of tubes 1-10, add 0.2 ml of the suspension of FII-coated latex as prepared in step 1. Shake the tubes thoroughly, and incubate at $56°C$ for 90 minutes. Allow the tubes to cool at room temperature, and incubate them overnight at $4°C$.

Slide Test

Materials

1. Latex-globulin reagent (RA-Test, Hyland)
2. Glycine-saline buffer diluent, pH 8.2 (RA-Test, Hyland)
3. RA serum and normal human serum
4. Microscope slides

Method

1. Prepare an approximate 1:20 dilution of the test serum by adding 1 drop of serum to 20 drops of the diluent.
2. Place 1 drop of the diluted serum onto a microscope slide.
3. Add 1 drop of the latex-globulin reagent to the diluted serum, mix with an applicator stick and spread over an area with a diameter of approximately 15 mm.
4. Tilt the slide from side to side and observe for macroscopic clumping.
    A. Negative: smooth suspension with no visible flocculation
    B. Weakly reactive: visible flocculation but with small aggregates or only partial clumping
    C. Reactive: visible flocculation with large aggregates and complete clumping (clear background). Visible flocculation usually occurs in a few seconds.

REFERENCES

1. Heller, G., Jacobson, A. S., Kolodny, M. H., and Kammerer, W. H. The hemagglutination test for rheumatoid arthritis. II. The influence of human plasma Fraction II (γ globulin) on the reaction. *J. Immunol. 72*, 66 (1954).
2. Rose, H. M., Ragan, C., Pearce, E., and Lipman, M. O. Differential agglutination of normal and sensitized sheep erythrocytes by sera of patients with rheumatoid arthritis. *Proc. Soc. Exptl. Biol. Med. 68*, 1 (1948).
3. Singer, J. M. and Plotz, C. M. The latex fixation test. I. Application to the serological diagnosis of rheumatoid arthritis. *Am. J. Med. 21*, 888 (1956).
4. Waaler, E. A factor in human serum activating the specific agglutination of sheep blood corpuscles. *Third Int'l Congress for Microbiol., New York, Abst. Commun.* (1939) p. 351.
5. Waller, M. V. and Vaughan, J. H. Use of anti-Rh sera for demonstrating agglutination activating factor in rheumatoid arthritis. *Proc. Soc. Exptl. Biol. Med. 92*, 198 (1956).

MIXED AGGLUTINATION WITH MONOLAYER CELL CULTURES

The principle of mixed agglutination was applied by Högman to monolayer cell cultures. In his experiments, cell cultures of human fetal cells were incubated with antisera to blood group A or B antigen. Thereafter a suspension of A or B erythrocytes was added. Adherence of A or B erythrocytes to the cell culture revealed the presence of A or B antigen on the cell surface. Högman's technique is capable of detecting only those antigens present on erythrocytes in addition to the cultured cells.

In order to overcome this limitation of Högman's technique, Fagraeus and Espmark introduced antiglobulin reagents into the indicator system. The indicator system with antiglobulin activity made the test more widely applicable to the study of cell surface antigens as well as their corresponding antibodies. By means of this technique, species specific and histocompatibility antigens have been demonstrated on cell cultures of various species.

Materials

1. Eight tubes with human HEp-2 cell cultures and eight tubes with murine-L cell cultures in metal racks (The tubes must be kept with the marked side up, since the cells are grown on the opposite side of glass wall.)
2. Rabbit antisera to human tissue and murine tissue and normal rabbit serum
3. 4% sheep-erythrocyte (SRBC) suspension
4. Rabbit antiserum to SRBC
5. Goat antiserum to rabbit γ globulins
6. LH medium (0.5% lactalbumin hydrolysate in Hanks' balanced salt solution) for antiserum dilution and final suspension of indicator erythrocytes
7. Phosphate buffered saline solution (PBS), pH 7.2
8. Test tubes, 10 x 75 mm
9. Pipettes, 1 ml and 5 ml

Method

1. Sensitization of cell cultures
    A. Set up one rack containing eight 10 x 75 mm tubes and label tubes as follows: $a_1, a_2, a_3, b_1, b_2, b_3, C, L$. Add 1.8 ml of LH medium to all tubes.
    B. Add 0.2 ml of a 1:10 dilution of rabbit anti-human-tissue serum to tube a_1 and mix well. Take a new pipette, and transfer 0.2 ml from tube a_1 to tube a_2, and mix well. Take a new pipette, and transfer 0.2 ml from tube a_2 to tube a_3, and mix well.

C. Repeat step 2 with the rabbit anti-murine-tissue serum using tubes b_1, b_2, and b_3.

D. Add 0.2 ml of a 1:10 dilution of normal rabbit serum to tube C, and mix well.

E. Label each row of cell culture tubes as follows:

$$\text{HEp-2 cells: } a_1, a_2, a_3, b_1, b_2, b_3, C, L$$
$$\text{L cells: } a_1, a_2, a_3, b_1, b_2, b_3, C, L$$

Remove stoppers from all culture tubes, and discard medium. Add 1.0 ml of LH medium to each tube, using automatic pipette; shake the rack gently to wash the monolayer surface; and discard medium. Repeat twice, and drain the culture tubes on a paper towel.

F. Take 1.0 ml from 10 x 75 mm tube L and add 0.5 ml to culture tube L of each cell line. Using the same pipette, take 1.0 ml from 10 x 75 mm tube C and add 0.5 ml to culture tube C of each cell line.

G. Take a new pipette, and transfer 0.5 ml of the anti-human-serum dilutions to the corresponding culture tubes, starting with the highest dilution, tube a_3.

H. Using a new pipette, repeat step 7 with the anti-murine-serum dilution, starting with tube b_3.

I. Close culture tubes with parafilm, and incubate the tubes, marked sides up, at room temperature for two hours.

2. Preparation of indicator erythrocytes

A. Put 1.0 ml of 4% sheep-erythrocyte suspension in a 16 x 100 mm tube, and add 1.0 ml of an appropriate (e.g. 1:4000) dilution of rabbit antiserum to sheep erythrocytes. Mix well and incubate the tube for 30 minutes at $37°C$.

B. Wash the sensitized erythrocytes three times with PBS, and resuspend in 2.0 ml of PBS.

C. Add 2.0 ml of 1:10 dilution of goat anti-rabbit-γ-globulin serum to the sensitized erythrocyte suspension, mix well, and incubate for 45 minutes at room temperature.

D. Wash the erythrocytes three times with PBS. Each time the erythrocytes must be resuspended thoroughly using a Pasteur pipette. Resuspend the indicator erythrocytes in 16 ml of LH medium, and keep the suspension in a 125-ml Erlenmeyer flask.

3. Incubation of cell cultures with indicator erythrocytes

A. After incubation of the cell cultures with the antiserum, discard the antiserum and wash the cell cultures three times with LH medium, following instructions given in section 1, step E.

B.   Shake the flask containing the indicator erythrocytes to obtain a homogeneous suspension. Add 0.5 ml of the indicator suspension to each culture tube, using a 50-ml pipette.

C.   Incubate the culture tubes for one hour at room temperature with the marked side up.

D.   After incubation, examine each cell-culture tube under a microscope at a low magnification for the binding of the indicator erythrocytes to the monolayer. Record the results in the protocol according to the following criteria:

+++: 80% or more of monolayer surface is covered by the indicator erythrocytes

++: 50 to 80% of monolayer surface is covered by the indicator erythrocytes

+: 20 to 50% of monolayer surface is covered by the indicator erythrocytes

—: No, or only a few, indicator erythrocytes are attached to the monolayer

Protocol 3.4.   Mixed Agglutination with Cell Cultures

| | Rabbit antiserum to: | | | | | | Controls NRS LH |
	Human tissues			Murine tissues			
Serum dilution	1:100	1:1000	1:10,000	1:100	1:1000	1:10,000	1:100
HEp-2 cells							
L cells							

REFERENCES

1.   Abeyounis, C. J., Milgrom, F., and Witebsky, E. Homotransplantation antibodies detected by mixed agglutination with cell culture monolayers.

Nature 203, 313 (1964).

2.   Coombs, R. R. A. and Franks, D. Immunological reactions involving two cell types. *Prog. in Allergy 13*, 174 (1969).

3.   Fagraeus, A. and Espmark, A. Use of a "mixed haemadsorption" method in virus-infected tissue cultures. *Nature 190*, 370 (1961).

4.   Högman, C. The principle of mixed agglutination applied to tissue culture systems: A method of study of cell-bound blood-group antigens. *Vox Sang. 4*, 12 (1959).

5.   Kano, K. and Milgrom, F. Nature of isoantibodies combining with human cell cultures. *Int. Arch. Aller. & Appl. Immunol. 31*, 209 (1967).

6.   McDonald, J. C., Milgrom, F., Abeyounis, C. J., and Witebsky, E. Mixed agglutination with cell cultures in rabbit homotransplantation. *Proc. Soc. Exptl. Biol. Med. 118*, 397 (1965).

7.   Milgrom, F., Kano K., Barron, A. L., and Witebsky, E. Mixed agglutination in tissue culture. *J. Immunol. 92*, 8 (1964).

8.   Milgrom, F., Kano, K., and Witebsky, E. The mixed agglutination test in studies on human transplantation. *J. A. M. A. 192*, 845 (1965).

9.   Milgrom, F., Abeyounis, C. J., McDonald, J. C., and Witebsky, E. Studies on antibodies accompanying homograft rejection. *Proc. Xth Intern. Soc. Blood Transf., Stockholm 1964, Bibl. Haemat. 23*, 155 (1965).

10. Wiener, A. S. and Herman, M. The second stage of the agglutination reaction. *J. Immunol. 36*, 255 (1939).

Chapter 4

IMMUNOHEMATOLOGIC PROCEDURES

J. F. Mohn   R. M. Lambert

Immunohematology is the oldest subspecialty of the discipline of immunology. Its origin can be traced to the fundamental observation made by Landois in 1875 that agglutination of the erythrocytes of one animal species usually occurred when they were mixed in vitro with the serum of another species. The basic concept embodied in this discovery was the inference that this hemagglutination was due to the presence of antigens on the red cell surface interacting with serum antibodies. Of almost equal importance, this finding established the species specificity of the erythrocytic elements of blood.

A quarter of a century later, Karl Landsteiner first noted a similar agglutination of human red blood cells by human sera, a totally intraspecies reaction. Based on the hemagglutination patterns he obtained in his crosshatch experiments, he could divide the blood of all humans into three distinct serologic groups, now known as the ABO blood groups. The fourth and rarest group in this system was discovered in 1902 by his pupils and associates, von Decastello and Sturli. Landsteiner was fully cognizant of the important role these blood group antigenic differences played in blood transfusion and used this information in laying the foundation for safe transfusion practice.

Perhaps of even greater importance than the practical application of this knowledge in reducing sharply the immunolgic hazard and thus establishing firmly the prospect of blood transfusion, this discovery of the human blood groups represents the origin of a new immunologic principle or antigenic system, called isospecificity (*isos*, Greek: equal). This is based on the existence of different antigens occurring within a single animal species, isoantigens, and their corresponding, specific antibodies, isoagglutinins, with their interaction resulting in the phenomenon of isoagglutination, which in the case of the blood groups is often referred to as isohemagglutination since erythrocytes are involved.

Acquired hemolytic anemia, more properly referred to in modern terminology as autoimmune hemolytic anemia, was the first human disease in which the involvement of an immunologic process or mechanism was implicated in its

71

pathogenesis. That this was possibly based on the development of autoantibodies was indicated from the time of the first observations of Widal, Abrami, and Brulé in 1908. These pioneers, who gave the first accurate descriptions of acquired hemolytic anemia, stressed that autoagglutination was characteristic of their cases.

Steadfastly maintaining its historic posture as a cardinal subdiscipline of immunology, immunohematology has developed in the past 70 years to such an extent that any attempt to embrace all of the procedures and their modifications currently employed in the diagnostic and investigative aspects of this field in the section allocated to this topic would be impossible. Consequently, only the primary, fundamental techniques of wide application in immunohematology will be presented.

REFERENCES

1. Dacie, J. V. *The Haemolytic Anaemias, Congenital and Acquired, Part II--The Auto-immune Haemolytic Anaemias*, 2nd ed. (J. & A. Churchill Ltd.: London, 1962).
2. Mohn, J. F. Blood Groups. In N. R. Rose, F. Milgrom, and C. J. van Oss, Eds., *Principles of Immunology* (The Macmillan Co.: New York, 1973), Chap. 25.
3. Race, R. R. and Sanger, R. *Blood Groups in Man*, 5th ed. (Blackwell Scientific Publications, Ltd.: Oxford, 1968).

DETERMINATION OF ABO AND Rh_0(D) BLOOD GROUPS

The extent of the blood grouping examination on patients and donors that is both reasonable and practical in preparation for blood transfusion poses somewhat of a problem to blood banks and transfusionists because of the increasing complexity of the red cell antigens and the vagaries of the reactions of the corresponding isoantibodies and their relative significance as applied to a transfusion service. Selection of appropriate tests demands distinctions between (1) the routine and the special case and (2) the donor and the recipient.

The only antigens for which donors and recipients should routinely be examined are A, B, and Rh_0(D).

In every instance, the ABO group must be determined by an examination of both the cell properties (agglutinogens) and the serum properties (agglutinins) with the single exception of infants up to the age of two to three months. In contrast to the readily detectable presence of these isoantigens at birth, only approximately 35 to 40% of newborn infants possess demonstrable isoagglutinins, which are all passively derived from the mother by transplacental filtration. Those present at birth regularly disappear from the infant's circulation, usually within the first seven to ten days of life. There then exists a hiatus lasting for two to three months, occasionally for as long as six months, when no antibodies at all may be found in the infant's serum. Thereafter, the child's own isoagglutinins are produced rapidly, rising in titer until the age of five to ten years. Serum examinations in this specific instance are unreliable and only the cellular antigens need to be determined. With respect to adults, however, serum antibody confirmation of the cell ABO group may be vital in preventing errors in the correct blood group identification of persons of subgroups of A and AB, especially group A_3B, or of weak variants of the A and B antigens. It is too often neglected in favor of tests for less clinically important red cell antigens or to save time. The complete ABO grouping based on the cell and serum characteristics is still the major blood group determination in transfusion practice.

All that is required for the Rh determination is a test with anti-D(Rh_0) serum. For transfusion purposes it is only necessary to know whether patients and blood donors are $Rh_0(D)$ positive or $Rh_0(D)$ negative. In Rh grouping the use of the terms $Rh_0(D)$ positive and $Rh_0(D)$ negative should be mandatory in place of Rh positive or Rh negative, too commonly used by many clinical services in referring to a person's Rh group. These awkward appearing and sounding designations are intended to emphasize specifically that this is the result of testing for precisely this clinically significant and routinely determined Rh antigen, the D antigen, also referred to as Rh_0 antigen, of the several now known to comprise the Rh system. The Rh symbol, instead of being replaced completely with the more sensible notation D, has been maintained out of the common usage that arose in medical practice from the early days when it was thought that Rh was but a single antigen.

There are distinct advantages to test tube centrifugation techniques over slide tests, and tube procedures are generally the method of choice of most workers for blood group determinations. Tubes are preferable to slides because: (a) they permit rapid reading of the results since agglutination can be greatly accelerated by centrifugation; (b) they allow for the detection of weak reactions that may occur, especially in the serum antibody confirmation of the ABO group, by bringing cells minimally sensitized with antibodies together at the bottom of the tube, permitting a lattice formation to occur; (c) tests made in tubes can be examined repeatedly over long periods of time if necessary; (d) the reaction mixtures can be incubated at any temperature in a waterbath or incubator; (e) there is no problem with drying of the reagents as only a minimum of evaporation is permitted with the small surface area of fluid; and (f) they can be used for large-scale work allowing many specimens of blood to be examined simultaneously. There is no justification for performing a slide test when equipment is available for the test tube technique.

The major disadvantage of slide tests is that the reagents dry rather rapidly with the resultant tendency for rouleaux formation to increase as evaporation takes place, thus permitting only a sharply restricted time for reading the agglutination. Consequently, slide tests are satisfactory only when confined to those antigen-antibody reactions known to occur by this method and when very potent antisera are available that are capable of producing visible agglutination within one or two minutes and maximum agglutination actively within five minutes of the cells and serum being mixed on the slide at room temperature. Again it should be emphasized that in the ABO serum confirmation tests, certain weak anti-A and anti-B agglutinins may not reach maximum activity with homologous cells within this time. $Rh_0(D)$ determinations using the slide technique, where warming boxes are required to raise the reaction temperature to the optimum of $37°C$, tend to promote even more rapid drying of the reaction mixture.

If blood specimens are received in an anticoagulant such as ACD or CPD solutions, it is essential that the red cells used in blood group determinations be washed free of their own plasma with saline solution at least once. If this is not carried out, clots can form when the red cells are mixed with the reagent antisera. With the slide method, if whole blood is mixed with antisera, any flakes of fibrin that form may be mistaken for agglutinates. Plasma also tends to cause rouleaux formation which can interfere with the interpretation of agglutination tests read macroscopically. Most important of all, irrespective of whether the sample contains an anticoagulant or is clotted blood, the plasma or serum contains soluble ABH blood group substances of the ABO system analogous to those on the erythrocytes when the individual is a secretor. These soluble substances have been known to inhibit the respective antibodies in the grouping antisera, aborting or abolishing the reaction with the corresponding antigenic receptors on the erythrocytes leading to a negative result. This neutralizing effect of serum substances has been especially reported in cases of pseudomucinous ovarian cysts.

Materials

1.   Blood, clotted (patient; donor; case)
2.   Anti-A serum
3.   Anti-B serum
4.   Anti-D serum (saline tube test)
5.   2% PBS suspensions of group A_1 $Rh_0(D)$ negative, group A_2 $Rh_0(D)$ positive, and group B $Rh_0(D)$ positive red cells (controls)

6.   0.9% phosphate-buffered saline solution, pH 7.4 (PBS)
7.   Applicators, wood, plain
8.   Tubes, centrifuge, round, polycarbonate, capacity 15 ml
9.   Tubes, centrifuge, conical, polycarbonate, capacity 15 ml
10. Pipette, capillary (Pasteur), disposable, length 5½ in.
11. Tubes, culture, without rim, 7 x 75 mm, 12 x 75 mm, and 12 x 100 mm

Method

1.   Rim clot gently with applicators to produce good, free-cell suspension in the serum.
2.   Decant the serum-cell suspension into properly prelabeled 15-ml round centrifuge tube.
3.   Centrifuge at 1345 g for 5 minutes (3600 rpm Sorvall Model CW-1, CP12-3 General Purpose Angle Rotor) or at 733 g for 10 minutes (2000 rpm Sorvall Model GLC-1, HL-4 Horizontal Rotor with no. 548 Omni-Carrier and no. 565 Stainless Steel Insert, 6-place).
4.   Using a Pasteur pipette, carefully remove the supernatant serum.
5.   Place 6 drops into a prelabeled 12 x 75 mm tube and the remainder in a prelabeled 12 x 100 mm tube.
6.   Cork the 12 x 75 mm tube tightly and inactivate the serum for 10 minutes in a 56°C waterbath.

Note: *The serum in the 12 x 100 mm tube, after being tightly stoppered, is stored active at 4°C for use in comparative tests or for preparing serum-cell suspensions for Rh genotyping with those antisera requiring a protein milieu.*

7.   Suspend the cells remaining in the round centrifuge tube in 10-12 ml of 0.9% phosphate-buffered saline solution (PBS).
8.   Centrifuge at 1345 g for 5 minutes or at 733 g for 10 minutes.
9.   Aspirate off the PBS wash-solution as completely as possible.
10. After resuspending the cells in 10-12 ml of 0.9% PBS, transfer the suspension to a properly prelabeled 15-ml conical centrifuge tube.
11. Centrifuge at 1345 g for 5 minutes or at 733 g for 10 minutes.
12. Aspirate off the PBS wash-solution as completely as possible.
13. Add sufficient 0.9% PBS to the packed cells to produce approximately a 2% suspension as visually compared to the accurately prepared 2% (v/v) suspensions of the control cells.
14. Label three rows of four 7 x 75 mm tubes Ia-Id, IIa-IId, and IIIa-IIId for the control cells, and one row of seven 7 x 75 mm tubes with the specimen

accession number plus a-g (e.g., 39a, 39b, 39c, etc.) for each case sample being examined.

15. Add 1 drop of antiserum, saline solution (PBS), or case serum to each tube in the horizontal rows according to the protocol as follows:

row a	anti-A serum
row b	anti-B serum
row c	anti-D serum
row d	0.9% PBS
row e	case serum
row f	case serum
row g	case serum

16. Add one drop of 2% cell suspensions to each tube in the vertical rows according to the protocol as follows:

row I	group A_1 $Rh_0(D)$ negative control cells
row II	group A_2 $Rh_0(D)$ positive control cells
row III	group B $Rh_0(D)$ positive control cells
row "specimen no."	case cells (from that specimen)

17. Add one drop of 2% serum-check cell suspensions to each tube in the horizontal rows (except where blocked out) according to the protocol as follows:

row e	group A_1
row f	group A_2
row g	group B

18. Mix by shaking the racks gently.
19. Incubate 15 minutes at room temperature.

Note: Most commercial producers of anti-D serum recommend incubation at 37°C for this reaction.

20. Centrifuge at 1200 g for 15 seconds (3600 rpm Sorvall Model CW-1, DA-12 Dual Angle Rotor) or at 275 g for 2 minutes (1215 rpm Sorvall Model GLC-1, HL-4 Horizontal Rotor with no. 548 Omni-Carrier and no. 590 Stainless Steel Insert, 40-place).
21. Examine each tube macroscopically for agglutination and record the results in Protocol 4.1.

Protocol 4.1.   Determination of ABO and Rh$_0$(D) Blood Groups

1 drop 2% saline (PBS) cell suspensions				
	Controls			Cases
Antisera	I	II	III	
1 drop	A$_1$	A$_2$	B	
	Rh$_0$(D)	Rh$_0$(D)	Rh$_0$(D)	
	neg	pos	pos	

(a) Anti-A

(b) Anti-B

(c) Anti-D

(d) Saline

1 drop undiluted case serum (inactivated)

(e) A$_1$
   cells
   1 drop

(f) A$_2$
   cells
   1 drop

(g) B
   cells
   1 drop

REFERENCES

1. Mohn, J. F. Blood Groups. In N. R. Rose, F. Milgrom, and C. J. van Oss, Eds., *Principles of Immunology* (The Macmillan Co.: New York, 1973), Chap. 25.
2. Mollison, P. L. *Blood Transfusion in Clinical Medicine*, 5th ed. (Blackwell Scientific Publications, Ltd.: Oxford, 1972), pp. 392, 399.
3. Race, R. R. and Sanger, R. *Blood Groups in Man*, 5th ed. (Blackwell Scientific Publications, Ltd.: Oxford, 1968), pp. 9, 171.
4. Stratton, F. and Renton, P. H. *Practical Blood Grouping* (Blackwell Scientific Publications, Ltd.: Oxford, 1958), p. 28.
5. M. M. Strumia, W. H. Crosby. J. G. Gibson, 2nd, T. J. Greenwalt, and J. R. Krevans, Eds., *General Principles of Blood Trasnfusions* (J. B. Lippincott Co.: Philadelphia, 1963). Published originally in *Transfusion 3*, 303 (1963).

DETERMINATION OF ABH SECRETOR STATUS

Many cells other than erythrocytes have been shown to contain the A and B antigens on their membranes; in fact, the cells of almost the entire body are stigmatized by the same blood group specific characteristics as the erythrocytes of the individual. Wide variation in concentrations exists in different organs, with the largest amounts being present in the submaxillary gland, esophagus, stomach, pancreas, and gall bladder; moderate amounts in the parotid gland, lung, liver, adrenal, and kidney; and trace amounts in the testis and spleen, for example. None has ever been detected in the brain, ocular lens, hair, compact bone, or cartilage.

Water-soluble A and B specific substances have been found in normal secretions such as saliva, gastric juice, bile, urine, amniotic fluid, and sweat, as well as in pathologic secretions such as pleural, pericardial, ascitic and hydrocele fluids, and pseudomucinous ovarian cyst fluid, an especially rich source with very high concentrations. On the other hand, they are never present in cerebrospinal fluid. They may be demonstrated in these body fluids by two techniques: (1) direct precipitation, a relatively insensitive method not applicable to routine testing since it requires very potent antisera such as rabbit antihuman erythrocyte heteroantisera or immune human isoantisera; and (2) specific inhibition of agglutination. Certain secretions of a group A person such as gastric juice, saliva, and semen, may contain enormous amounts of A antigen in comparison with the A activity demonstrable on erythrocytes as measured by the absorption capacity of a 50% suspension of human group A_1 red cells.

This phenomenon of secretion is an inherited characteristic under the direct control of a pair of allelic Mendelian genes, *Se*, the secretor gene, and *se*, the nonsecretor gene. Without exception, the *Se* gene is dominant to the *se* gene and when present either in the homozygous or heterozygous state conveys the ability to secrete either A or B water-soluble substance depending upon the individual's ABO group. Consequently, persons of the genotypes *SeSe* and *Sese* are secretors. Nonsecretors represent the homozygous state *sese* genotype. This represents an independent gene system with no linkage to the ABO genes, an instance of genetic independence yet with intimate association. All population groups examined in Europe and America have shown the frequency of secretors to be 77 to 78% and that of nonsecretors 22 to 23%. The only known exceptions are North American Indians and Australian aborigines.

The A and B antigens exist in two distinct forms: (1) Alcohol-soluble: glycolipid. The membrane antigens present in all tissues and on erythrocytes with the exception of the brain and in all persons, whether secretors or nonsecretors, are of this variety. It is not present in secretions and is not influenced by the *Se* gene. (2) Water-soluble: polysaccharide. This is easily extracted from the tissues of secretors but does not occur in aqueous extracts of the organs of nonsecretors. It is not on the red blood cells and its presence in most body fluids of secretors except for the spinal fluid is determined by the *Se* gene. The largest quantities are found in glandular organs, the concentrations closely paralleling those in the corresponding secretions.

Since the alcohol-soluble substances are not under control of the secretor genes, the erythrocytes and tissues of both secretors and nonsecretors are stigmatized by the A and B glycolipids. Therefore, examinations of the erythrocyte properties in determinations of the ABO group are reliable since they are not affected by the secretor status of the individual.

Certain carefully selected, normal, bovine sera when properly absorbed with human group A_1 or A_1B erythrocytes were shown by Schiff in 1927 to agglutinate selectively human group O red blood cells. In addition, he proved that this heteroagglutination reaction was specifically inhibited by human saliva or group O secretors. Extensive studies by many investigators clearly indicated that such bovine sera did not contain true "anti-O" agglutinins detecting a specific receptor on human erythrocytes that was the direct product of the *O* gene because the characteristic pattern of reactions, if these antibodies were specific for group O, was not obtained. For example, repeated absorptions of bovine sera with human group AB cells removed all the "anti-O" activity.

In 1941 Witebsky and Klendshoj demonstrated unequivocally that isolated, purified polysaccharide from the gastric juice of human group AB secretors exhibited an O inhibitory activity in addition to the expected A and B, although a group AB person cannot possess an O gene. Similarly, they found that substances isolated from human group A and group B secretor salivas inhibited the agglutination of human group O erythrocytes by absorbed bovine "anti-O" antisera to the same extent as O substance extracted from human gastric juice of group O secretors. On the contrary, this so-called "O" substance did not inhibit the agglutination of human group A cells by anti-A sera or group B cells by anti-B sera.

Based on a comparison of many human and animal "anti-O" sera examined in inhibition tests with saliva specimens of human group O secretors, Morgan and Watkins reported in 1948 that they were able to divide such antisera into two distinct groups. Those that were inhibited by the substances tested were designated anti-H sera. As these antisera were neutralized by secretor salivas of any ABO group, they proposed that the inhibiting substance be correspondingly designated H substance for heterogenetic to indicate its ubiquitous nature, to emphasize it was not a product of the O gene, and to establish that it was immunologically distinct from any erythrocytic substance reacting with true anti-O antibodies. They felt this was a basic or primary substance common to all erythrocytes irrespective of the ABO groups. The remaining antisera were termed "anti-O" since they were uninfluenced by H substance in their action on group O erythrocytes. This postulation of a basic relationship of H substance to the A, B, and O agglutinogens, together with several cardinal discoveries made in the intervening years by other investigators, led Watkins and Morgan in 1959 to propose their scheme for the biosynthesis of the ABO blood group antigens. In this hypothesis, H substance, a product resulting from the action of an H gene, was considered to be the substrate that is catalytically transformed to A substance or B substance or both by specific enzymes under the control of either the A gene or B gene, if present. As this is only a partial conversion, the body fluids of all secretors contain H substance in addition to A or B substance.

The specific inhibition of agglutination technique is one of the most sensitive serologic tools available to the immunologist. It is exceptionally well suited to the demonstration of ABH substances in body fluids and saline extracts of tissues and can be designed to detect 0.00025 to 0.0005 μg quantities, especially if naturally-occurring or nonimmune human anti-A or anti-B sera are used. Saliva is the body fluid of choice for use in the determination of the secretor status of an individual because it contains large amounts of these blood group substances and is readily accessible. It is the key to secretion, for this is an all or nothing phenomenon. If the substances are absent from saliva they will be absent from the other secretions as well.

It is absloutely essential that saliva specimens be collected and processed properly and rapidly, as outlined below. This is requisite because the saliva of both secretors and nonsecretors contains bacterial enzymes produced chiefly by microorganisms of the family *Bacillaceae* that are capable of decomposing the ABH substances. Some of these are utterly specific for either the A, B, or H substances. The most important step, therefore, in processing the saliva is heating it to 100°C to inactivate these enzymes.

On the same day that the inhibition of agglutination experiment is to be carried out, a preliminary titration of the antiserum to be inhibited must be performed with the test cell suspension that will be used to determine the appropriate, minimum concentration of antibodies that will allow the maximum detection of minimum amounts of secreted substances. For the greatest sensitivity, a dilution of the antiserum should be selected that produces a firm but less than maximum agglutination of the test cells.

Since H substance is present in the saliva of all secretors irrespective of their ABO group, a single test system using an H antigen-anti-H reaction can be used in determining the secretor status of an individual. Neither naturally-occurring nor immune animal anti-H sera are readily available. In addition, they require preliminary absorption to remove the human species agglutinins. For this determination, therefore, anti-H lectin is preferred and readily obtainable. The most frequently used, potent, and reliable of the several known to exist is a saline extract of the seeds of *Ulex europaeus*, common gorse.

Materials

1. Saliva, undiluted, boiled (patient; case)
2. Anti-H lectin (*Ulex europaeus* seed extract)
3. 3% PBS suspension of group O red cells
4. Saliva of group O secretor, undiluted, boiled (control)
5. Saliva of group O nonsecretor, undiluted, boiled (control)
6. 0.9% phosphate-buffered saline solution, pH 7.4 (PBS)
7. Beaker, polyethylene, 50 ml
8. Tubes, screw-cap, polystyrene, 13 x 100 mm, capacity 8 ml
9. Tubes, centrifuge, conical, polycarbonate, capacity 15 ml
10. Tubes, culture, without rim, 10 x 75 mm, 12 x 75 mm, and 16 x 125 mm
11. Tube closures, stainless steel, Morton, 16 mm
12. Pipette, capillary (Pasteur), disposable, length 5½ in.
13. Pipette, serologic, 1.0 ml divided in 1/100
14. Pipette, serologic, 10.0 ml divided in 1/10

Method

1. Saliva preparation
    A. Collect specimen not less than 2 hours after a meal.
    B. Request donor to rinse mouth thoroughly with tap water at least 3 times no later than 10 minutes before collection begins and after

removing any dental prosthetic devices which might contain trapped food particles.

Note: For critical saliva examinations, the donor should also brush his teeth using a toothbrush moistened with tap water only.

C.   Collect the total volume of saliva secreted over a 30-minute period in a prelabeled 50-ml polyethylene beaker, recommending that the donor chew gently on the buccal mucosa or use any psychologic suggestion known to increase salivation.

Note: Do not use paraffin, gum, candy, or salivatory drugs to stimulate saliva flow.

D.   Transfer the entire amount of native, whole saliva to one or more prelabeled polystyrene, screw-cap tubes and cap them tightly.
E.   Freeze immediately at −25°C to −30°C overnight.

Note: A minimum storage period of 4 hours at −25°C will be satisfactory provided the whole saliva has really been frozen solidly for this time. Do not freeze or store on dry ice with these plastic tubes.

F.   Thaw the frozen saliva in a 37°C waterbath until it is just completely liquefied.
G.   Transfer the saliva at once to a prelabeled 15-ml conical centrifuge tube.
H.   Centrifuge at 3440 g for 20 minutes at 4°C (5000 rpm Sorvall Model RC-3, SP/X Rotor).
I.   Promptly remove the supernatant saliva using a 10.0-ml serologic pipette being careful not to disturb the sediment.

Note: The last amounts may have to be removed with a capillary pipette. If the centrifugation has been adequate and the sediment is firmly packed, it may be possible to effect this transfer by decanting.

J.   Transfer the supernatant to a 16 x 125 mm tube (glass) and cap with a Morton stainless-steel tube closure.
K.   Place the tube in a boiling waterbath and observe the saliva for signs of boiling as indicated by a steady stream of bubbles rising to the surface or the formation of a light-blue haze or opalescence.
L.   Boil the saliva for exactly 90 seconds.
M.   Remove the tube and put in the refrigerator at 4°C until cool enough

to handle, or cool under running tap water.

N.   Transfer the inactivated saliva to a prelabeled 15-ml conical centrifuge tube.

O.   Centrifuge at 3440 g for 20 minutes at 4°C.

Note: *For extreme clarification of the saliva in critical examinations, centrifuge at 12,100 g for 20 minutes (10,000 rpm Sorvall Model RC-2B, SS-1 Rotor).*

P.   Carefully remove the supernatant saliva using a 10.0-ml serologic pipette and a capillary pipette for the last amounts.

Q.   Place in an appropriate-size serum bottle with rubber-sleeve stopper, label properly, and freeze at −25° to −30°C until examined.

2.   Preliminary titration of lectin (Part I)

A.   Label twelve 10 x 75 mm tubes a1, a2, a3, and so on, to a12.

B.   Place 0.1 ml of 0.9% PBS into each of tubes a2-a12 with a 1.0-ml serologic pipette.

C.   Add 0.1 ml of anti-H lectin to each of tubes a1 and a2 with a 1.0-ml serologic pipette.

D.   Titrate lectin by preparing serial twofold dilutions in tubes a2-a11 by mixing contents of each tube in and out of the pipette 6 times, finally removing 0.1 ml of the dilution and transferring it to the next tube in sequence.

E.   Remove 0.1 ml from tube a11 and discard with the pipette.

F.   Add 0.1 ml of 0.9% PBS to each of tubes a1-a12.

G.   Shake rack gently to mix contents of tubes.

H.   Add 0.1 ml of 3% suspension of group O cells to each of tubes a1-a12.

I.   Shake rack gently to mix contents of tubes.

J.   Incubate at room temperature for 15 minutes.

K.   Centrifuge tubes at 600 g for 3 minutes (1800 rpm Sorvall Model GLC-1, HL-4 Horizontal Rotor with no. 548 Omni-Carrier and no. 575 Stainless Steel Insert, 20-place) or at 1200 g for 1 minute (3600 rpm Sorvall Model CW-1, DA-12 Dual Angle Rotor).

L.   Examine each tube macroscopically for agglutination and record the results in Protocol 4.2 according to the scheme listed following Protocol 4.3.

3.   Inhibition of agglutination (Part II)

A.   Select from the anti-H lectin titration the highest dilution yielding a +++(+) to ++++ reaction.

B.   Prepare a sufficient volume of this dilution of lectin for the inhibition test, considering the number of tubes involved.

C. Label 3 rows of twelve 10 x 75 mm tubes a1-a12, b1-b12, and c1-c12.
D. Place 0.1 ml of 0.9% PBS into each of tubes a2-a12, b2-b12, and c2-c12.
E. Add 0.1 ml of group O secretor saliva (control) to each of tubes a1 and a2.
F. Titrate saliva by preparing serial twofold dilutions in tubes a2-a11.
G. Remove 0.1 ml from tube a11 and discard with the pipette.
H. Repeat the procedure (steps D-G) in row b with the group O nonsecretor saliva (control)
I. Repeat the procedure (steps D-G) in row c with the unknown saliva (patient; case).
J. Add 0.1 ml of diluted anti-H lectin to each of tubes a1-a12, b1-b12, and c1-c12.
K. Shake racks gently to mix contents of tubes.

Protocol 4.2.   Preliminary Titration of Anti-H Lectin (Part I)

0.1 ml PBS + 0.1 ml 3% saline (PBS) group O cell suspension	
Anti-H lectin 0.1 ml	group O cells
(1) Undil	
(2) 1:2	
(3) 1:4	
(4) 1:8	
(5) 1:16	
(6) 1:32	
(7) 1:64	
(8) 1:128	
(9) 1:256	
(10) 1:512	
(11) 1:1024	
(12) Saline	

Protocol 4.3.   Inhibition of Agglutination (Part II)

0.1 ml 1:   dil. anti-H lectin + 0.1 ml 3% saline (PBS) group O cell suspension

---

Saliva i.a. 0.1 ml	group O sec. control a	group O sec. control b	c
(1) Undil			
(2) 1:2			
(3) 1:4			
(4) 1:8			
(5) 1:16			
(6) 1:32			
(7) 1:64			
(8) 1:128			
(9) 1:256			
(10) 1:512			
(11) 1:1024			
(12) Saline			

—	=	No agglutination (score 0)
±	=	Doubtful agglutination (score 0)
(+)	=	Trace agglutination; few fine agglutinates involving less that 50% of cells (score 1)
+	=	Slight agglutination; many fine agglutinates with no free cells (score 2)
++	=	Moderate agglutination; several (10-15) small to medium agglutinates with no free cells (score 4)
+++	=	Strong agglutination; few (3-5) large agglutinates with no free cells (score 6)
++++	=	Very strong agglutination (maximum); one solid clump of cells (score 8)

L.   Incubate at room temperature for 15 minutes.
M.   Add 0.1 ml of 3% suspension of group O cells to each of tubes a1-a12, b1-b12, and c1-c12.
N.   Shake racks gently to mix contents of tubes.
O.   Incubate at room temperature for 15 minutes.
P.   Centrifuge tubes at 600 g for 3 minutes or at 1200 g for 1 minute.
Q.   Examine each tube macroscopically for agglutination and record the results in Protocol 4.3 according to the scheme following it.

REFERENCES

1.   Hartmann, G. *Group Antigens in Human Organs* (Ejnar Mundsgaard Forlag: Copenhagen, 1941). Reprinted in F. R. Camp and F. R. Ellis, Eds., *Selected Contributions to the Literature of Blood Groups and Immunology* (Blood Transfusion Division, U. S. Army Medical Research Laboratory: Fort Knox, Ky., 1970).
2.   Kabat, E. A. *Blood Group Substances* (Academic: New York, 1956).
3.   Morgan, W. T. J. and Watkins, W. M. The detection of a product of the blood group *O* gene and the relationship of the so-called O-substance to the agglutinogens A and B. *Brit. J. Exptl. Pathol. 29*, 159 (1948).
4.   Race, R. R. and Sanger R. *Blood Groups in Man*, 5th ed., (Blackwell Scientific Publications, Ltd.: Oxford, 1968), pp. 39, 61, 291.
5.   Watkins, W. M. and Morgan, W. T. J. Possible genetical pathways for the biosynthesis of blood group mucopolysaccharides. *Vox Sang. 4*, 97 (1959).
6.   Witebsky, E. and Klendshoj, N. C. The isolation of an O specific substance from gastric juice of secretors and carbohydrate-like substances from gastric juice of non-secretors. *J. Exptl. Med. 73*, 655 (1941).

DETECTION OF INCOMPLETE ANTI-D ANTIBODIES

Based on their determinations of the Rh groups and detection of anti-Rh antibodies in an extensive examination of 350 cases, Levine and his collaborators demonstrated that hemolytic disease of the newborn was directly related to fetomaternal Rh incompatibility and that isoimmunization of pregnancy was the cause of this disease in which the Rh blood group system is very often involved. It was fortuitous that Levine and his co-workers were able to demonstrate antibodies in vitro in their initial cases by using the classical serologic milieu of saline solution. Subsequently other investigators were not able to detect agglutinins in the maternal sera by this customary technique in more than 50% of their cases, even though they were quite typical examples of hemolytic disease of the newborn with 100% showing the clinical, hematologic, biochemical, and pathologic signs in the newborn and the expected Rh groups of the mother and father.

This apparent discordancy with Levine's theory of the pathogenesis of hemolytic disease of the newborn was eliminated by the almost simultaneous, independent finding of a new variety of anti-Rh antibodies by Race and Wiener in 1944. They introduced the terms incomplete and blocking, respectively, to refer to the kind of Rh antibodies that combined with D positive erythrocytes, but failed to agglutinate them when the reactions were performed conventionally in saline solution. The term incomplete antibody implied there was something deficient about the integrity of the normal, complete antibody molecule. The term blocking antibody was designed to describe the observation that the nonagglutinating antibodies, by coating the red blood cells, could inhibit or block the agglutination of these cells by saline-active, complete antibodies. The indirect procedure they reported for detecting these antibodies was cumbersome to perform and not too sensitive in that it revealed antibodies in at most only 60% of those maternal sera that were nonreactive in saline solution.

A more efficient and reliable technique came into routine use when Diamond and Abelson found that incomplete anti-D antibodies would cause agglutination directly if the undiluted maternal serum being examined for the presence of antibodies was reacted on a slide with D positive erythrocytes suspended in their own serum or plasma. This led to the substitution of human group AB serum for saline solution as a diluent for titrating the maternal serum under investigation and for suspending the D positive test cells in test tube procedures. Following the observation made by Diamond and Denton, human group AB serum (or other ABO compatible serum) was replaced by 20% bovine serum albumin solution, which proved to be more effective and could be made readily available in large volumes. The best all-protein diluent for this purpose has been shown to be a mixture of equal parts of undiluted, human group AB serum (or other ABO compatible serum) and 30% bovine serum albumin solution. Synthetic preparations such as dextran and polyvinylpyrrolidone (PVP) have also been used but to a much lesser extent.

In 1945 Coombs, Mourant, and Race described their indirect antiglobulin technique for demonstrating Rh antibodies in those sera containing only the incomplete variety. In this test advantage is taken of the fact that these incomplete antibodies do accomplish the first phase of agglutination, specifically unite with the D antigenic receptor sites on the erythrocytes, commonly expressed as coating or sensitizing the cells, and that this antigen-antibody union will withstand several washes with saline solution to remove the other serum proteins. The presence of these antibody molecules on the red cell surface is then determined by the addition of rabbit, goat, or sheep antihuman globulin serum which bridges the gap between the incomplete Rh antibody-sensitized cells allowing a lattice formation with subsequent agglutination. This technique is an invaluable addition to the serologist's armamentarium and is extremely useful for the detection of most incomplete blood group antibodies irrespective of the antigen-antibody system involved.

Following the observation made in 1946 by Pickles that treatment of D positive erythrocytes with the enzymes present in a bacterial-free filtrate of a broth culture of cholera vibrio (*Vibrio comma*) rendered those red cells agglutinable by incomplete anti-D antibodies in saline solution, Morton and Pickles found that trypsin produced the same effect. Since that time it has been shown that mild pretreatment of D positive red cells with various enzymes, especially trypsin, papain, ficin, and bromelin, is extremely effective in allowing the incomplete antibodies to produce direct agglutination of such treated test cells in saline solution.

Anti-Rh antibodies may belong either to the IgM or the IgG immunoglobulin class. The saline-active, complete anti-Rh agglutinins were shown by ultracentrifugal analysis to have a sedimentation constant of 19 S and by electrophoretic migration to be the relatively large IgM globulins; the albumin-active, incomplete antibodies similarly were shown to have a sedimentation constant of 7 S and to be the smaller IgG globulins. It is now clear that the inability of the incomplete IgG antibodies to agglutinate cells suspended in saline solution is directly related to their small size and the resultant inability to span the distance between erythrocytes in suspension. Concerning their pathogenetic role in hemolytic disease of the newborn, only the IgG antibodies are significant, since they alone can traverse the placental barrier and enter the circulation of the fetus. It is a frequent occurrence in isoimmunization to fetal erythrocytic D antigens to observe that saline-active, or IgM, agglutinins appear in the maternal serum early in the pregnancy to disappear and be replaced by albumin-active, or IgG, antibodies as the pregnancy proceeds to term.

According to Pollack et al., the ability of proteins and other macromolecules to support agglutination by incomplete IgG anti-Rh antibodies depends on their respective dielectric constants or capacity to dissipate the cloud of cations surrounding the negatively charged red cell membrane and thereby reducing the zeta potential between the two charged layers. Since the zeta potential represents the repulsive force keeping erythrocytes separated from one another, an appropriate reduction in this force will permit the cells to come sufficiently close together to be agglutinated by the small IgG antibodies. Brooks and Seaman, however, point out that the dielectric effect measured by Pollack for dextran most definitely cannot have the influence he attributed to it. According to van Oss, the adsorption of the polymers on the cell surfaces may cause aggregation by polymer bridging.

The antiglobulin reaction overcomes the separation of the cells by physically bridging the distance between the IgG antibody-coated cells with heteroantibodies to the human IgG antibody molecules. This result is analogous to extending the length of the IgG antibody molecules to approximately that of the IgM antibody molecules which are capable of reaching across this distance on their own because of their inherent length.

Although the enzymes commonly used in blood group serology for this purpose are noted for their proteolytic properties, their major role in this instance appears to be the reduction of the negative charges on the erythrocyte surface resulting in a decrease in the zeta potential. Since the surface charge is primarily due to the carboxyl groups of sialic acid, the liberation of sialomucopeptides containing N-acetyl neuraminic acid by trypsin and neuraminidase diminishes this charge, raises the isoelectric point and renders the cells more agglutinable by incomplete antibodies. As Pollack et al. view it, this change in surface negative charges causes a concomitant change in the cloud of positive charges in the environment surrounding the cells.

The presumption that the only effect of enzyme treatment of red cells is to reduce their surface negative charges may not be entirely correct. It has been shown by van Oss and Mohn that papain also distorts the shape of the erythrocyte tending to produce a spherical and irregularly shaped cell. The protrusions produced by this treatment probably allow cellular contact with resultant agglutination as described by van Oss, Gillman, and Good for phagocytes.

The primary usefulness of enzyme-treatment of erythrocytes in blood group immunology has been to increase the sensitivity of agglutination reactions and especially to convert incomplete or nonagglutinating blood group antibody-antigen reactions to those that readily result in agglutination in saline solution. Although enzyme pretreatment enhances the agglutination of erythrocytes by many blood group antibodies, the blood group MN and Fy (Duffy) red cell receptors are destroyed. It is appropriate, therefore, to use enzymes in addition to other methods in the serologic characterization of known blood group antibodies and antigens. Enzymes are valuable in blood group determinations only when the reagent antisera have been thoroughly studied serologically.

One-stage enzyme techniques in which test cells, antiserum, and enzyme solution are mixed together simultaneously suffer from the potential destruction of some of the antibodies. Two-stage procedures in which test cells are treated with enzyme solution and then washed before the addition of antiserum are generally preferred for this reason.

Enzyme Treatment of Erythrocytes

Materials

1. $Rh_0(D)$ positive ($R_1 R_1$ or $R_2 R_2$) group O blood, in ACD solution
2.   0.1% ficin solution in Hendry's buffer, pH 7.4
3.   Hendry's buffer solution, pH 7.4
4.   0.9% phosphate-buffered saline solution, pH 7.4 (PBS)
5.   Flask, Erlenmeyer, 25 ml
6.   Tubes, centrifuge, round, polycarbonate, capacity 15 ml
7.   Tubes, centrifuge, conical, polycarbonate, capacity 15 ml
8.   Pipette, serologic, 5.0 ml divided in 1/10
9.   Pipette, serologic, 0.2 ml divided in 1/100
10. Tissues, disposable, Kimwipes

Method

1.   Gently mix the $Rh_0(D)$ positive whole ACD blood by inverting sufficient times to resuspend the cells completely in the plasma.
2.   With a 5.0-ml serologic pipette, remove 2.0 ml of ACD blood using the last 2.0-ml divisions of the pipette.
3.   Expel the blood into approximately 10 ml of 0.9% phosphate-buffered saline solution (PBS) in a 15-ml round centrifuge tube and mix well by drawing the saline-blood suspension in and blowing it out of the pipette gently several times.
4.   Centrifuge at 1345 g for 5 minutes (3600 rpm Sorvall Model CW-1, CP12-3 General Purpose Angle Rotor) or at 733 g for 10 minutes (2000 rpm Sorvall Model GLC-1, HL-4 Horizontal Rotor with no. 548 Omni-Carrier and no. 565 Stainless Steel Insert, 6-place).
5.   Aspirate off the PBS wash-solution as completely as possible.
6.   Suspend the cells remaining in the round centrifuge tube in 10-12 ml of 0.9% PBS.
7.   Repeat steps 4-6 two more times for a total of three washes.
8.   Aspirate off the PBS wash-solution as completely as possible.
9.   After resuspending the cells in 10-12 ml of 0.9% PBS, transfer the suspension to a 15-ml conical centrifuge tube.
10. Centrifuge at 1345 g for 5 minutes or at 733 g for 10 minutes.
11. Aspirate off the PBS wash-solution as completely as possible.
12. With a 0.2-ml serologic pipette remove exactly 0.2 ml of packed red cells, inserting the tip of the pipette well below the upper, saline-diluted layer of cells before drawing cells up into the pipette, and carefully wipe off the

exterior of the pipette with a tissue.

13. Expel the packed cells into 4.8 ml of 0.1% ficin solution in a 25-ml Erlenmeyer flask, mix well by drawing the saline cell suspension in and blowing it out of the pipette gently several times, and stopper the flask.

Note: *This results in a 4% red cell suspension in 0.1% ficin solution.*

14. Incubate 10 minutes in a 37°C waterbath shaking gently at intervals to resuspend the cells.
15. Add approximately 5 ml of cold (4°C) 0.9% PBS to stop the digestion and mix well.
16. Transfer the cell suspension to a 15-ml round centrifuge tube.
17. Centrifuge at 1345 g for 5 minutes or at 733 g for 10 minutes.
18. Aspirate off the PBS wash-solution as completely as possible.
19. Resuspend the cells in 10-12 ml of cold (4°C) 0.9% PBS.
20. Repeat steps 17-19 two more times for a total of three washes.
21. After resuspending the cells in 10-12 ml of 0.9% PBS, transfer the suspension to a 15-ml conical centrifuge tube.
22. Centrifuge at 1345 g for 5 minutes or at 733 g for 10 minutes.
23. Aspirate off the PBS wash-solution as completely as possible.

Serologic Titration

Materials

1. Maternal serum, anti-D, undiluted, active
2. 2% suspensions of Rh_0(D) positive ($R_1 R_1$ or $R_2 R_2$) group O red cells in:
   (a) phosphate-buffered saline solution (PBS)
   (b) human serum+bovine albumin mixture
3. 2% PBS suspension of enzyme-treated Rh_0(D) positive group O red cells
4. 3% PBS suspension of Rh_0(D) positive group O red cells
5. 0.9% phosphate-buffered saline solution, pH 7.4 (PBS)
6. Human serum+bovine albumin mixture of equal parts group AB, undiluted, normal, native, adult, human serum and 30% bovine serum albumin.
7. Pipette, serologic, 1.0 ml divided in 1/100
8. Tubes, culture, without rim, 10 x 75 mm and 12 x 75 mm
9. Centrifuge, Sorvall Cell Washing, Model CW-1 with DA-12 Dual Angle Rotor
10. Automatic Filling Unit, Sorvall Model AF-2
11. Antihuman globulin serum (rabbit) (Coombs reagent)

Method

1. Label 4 rows of twelve 10 x 75 mm tubes a1-a12, b1-b12, c1-c12, and d1-d12.
2. Label one row of ten 12 x 75 mm tubes 2-11 for the master titration of the anti-D serum in 0.9% PBS.
3. Add 0.9% PBS as follows:
    (a) tubes 2-11 (master titration):   0.4 ml
    (b) tubes a12, b12, and c12:   0.1 ml
4. Add anti-D serum as follows:
    (a) tubes a1, b1, and c1:   0.1 ml
    (b) tube 2 (master titration):   0.4 ml
5. Titrate anti-D serum in master titration row by mixing well contents of tube 2 in and out of the pipette 6 times.
6. Remove 0.7 ml from tube 2 and place 0.1 ml in each of tubes a2, b2, and c2 and 0.4 ml in tube 3 (master titration).
7. Continue this procedure until tube 11 is reached.
8. Remove 0.7 ml from tube 11 and place 0.1 ml in each of tubes a11, b11, and c11 and discard remaining with the pipette.
9. Place 0.1 ml of serum+albumin mixture into each of tubes d2-d12.
10. Add 0.1 ml of anti-D serum to each of tubes d1 and d2.
11. Titrate anti-D serum in serum+albumin by preparing serial twofold dilutions in tubes d2-d11 by mixing contents of each tube in and out of the pipette 6 times, finally removing 0.1 ml of the dilution and transferring it to the next tube in sequence.
12. Remove 0.1 ml from tube d11 and discard with the pipette.
13. With separate 1.0-ml serologic pipettes, add 0.1 ml of $Rh_0(D)$ positive cell suspensions to each tube as follows:
    (a) tubes a1-a12:   2% PBS suspension
    (b) tubes b1-b12:   2% PBS suspension of enzyme-treated cells
    (c) tubes c1-c12:   3% PBS suspension
    (d) tubes d1-d12:   2% serum+albumin suspension
14. Shake racks gently to mix contents of tubes.
15. Incubate 30 minutes in a 37°C waterbath.
16. Centrifuge tubes of rows a, b, and d at 600 g for 3 minutes (1800 rpm Sorvall Model GLC-1, HL-4 Horizontal Rotor with no. 548 Omni-Carrier and no. 575 Stainless Steel Insert, 20-place) or at 1200 g for 1 minute (3600 rpm Sorvall Model CW-1, DA-12 Dual Angle Rotor).
17. Reincubate tubes of rows a, b, and d for 5 minutes in a 37°C waterbath before reading directly from the waterbath.
18. Examine each tube macroscopically for agglutination and record the results

in Protocol 4.4.

19. Place tubes of row c in centrifuge rotor (DA-12, Dual Angle Rotor).
20. Place the distributor manifold over the rotor knob and rotate until the three pins engage in the three holes in the rotor making certain the distributor is flush with the rotor.
21. Mount rotor by fitting it over the motor shaft and engaging the holes in the bottom plate of the rotor onto the pins of the rotating centrifuge bowl.
22. Close centrifuge cover making certain the cover latch is securely fastened.
23. Turn CW-1 centrifuge cycle selector to "Auto."
24. Turn AF-2 filling unit wash cycle selector to "4."
25. Press signal button on AF-2 filling unit.
26. When buzzer sounds, remove rotor from centrifuge and take off distributor manifold.

Protocol 4.4.   Detection of Incomplete Anti-D Antibodies

0.1 ml 2% or 3% CDe/Ce($R_1 R_1$) group O cell suspensions				
Anti-D serum 0.1 ml	Saline a	Ficin-cells in saline b	Indirect antiglobulin c	Serum+ albumin d
(1) Undil				
(2) 1:2				
(3) 1:4				
(4) 1:8				
(5) 1:16				
(6) 1:32				
(7) 1:64				
(8) 1:128				
(9) 1:256				
(10) 1:512				
(11) 1:1024				
(12) Diluent				

27. Shake rotor gently to dislodge cell sediments.
28. Add 2 drops of antihuman globulin serum (Coombs reagent) to each tube.
29. Shake rotor gently to mix contents at once.
30. Reinsert rotor rapidly into centrifuge and close centrifuge cover.
31. Turn CW-1 centrifuge cycle selector to "Low" on left or Auto side of dial at once.
32. Turn timer to 60 seconds immediately.

Note: Centrifuge will run at 130 g for 60 seconds (1150-1200 rpm Sorvall Model CW-1).

33. Without delay, examine each tube macroscopically for agglutination and record the results in Protocol 4.4.

REFERENCES

1. Brooks, D. E. and Seaman, G. V. F. The effect of neutral polymers on the electrokinetic potential of cells and other charged particles. I. Models for the zeta potential increase. *J. Colloid Interf. Sci.* (in press).
2. Coombs, R. R. A., Mourant, A. E., and Race, R. R. A new test for the detection of weak and "incomplete" Rh agglutinins. *Brit. J. Exptl. Path.* 26, 255 (1945).
3. Diamond, L. K. and Abelson, N. M. The demonstration of anti-Rh agglutinins--an accurate and rapid slide test. *J. Lab. Clin. Med.* 30, 204 (1945).
4. Diamond, L. K. and Denton, R. L. Rh agglutination in various media with particular reference to the value of albumin. *J. Lab. Clin. Med.* 30, 821 (1945).
5. Lewis, A. J. Papain, ficin and bromelain in the detection of incomplete Rhesus antibodies. *Brit. J. Haematol.*, III, 332 (1957).
6. Mohn, J. F. Blood Groups. In N. R. Rose, F. Milgrom, and C. J. van Oss, Eds., *Principles of Immunology* (The Macmillan Co.: New York, 1973), Chap. 25.
7. Mollison, P. L. *Blood Transfusion in Clinical Medicine*, 5th ed. (Blackwell Scientific Publications, Ltd.: Oxford, 1972), pp. 202, 401.
8. Morton, J. A. and Pickles, M. M. Use of trypsin in the detection of incomplete anti-Rh antibodies. *Nature 159*, 779 (1947).
9. van Oss, C. J. Precipitation and Agglutination. In N. R. Rose, F. Milgrom, and C. J. van Oss, Eds., *Principles of Immunology* (The Macmillan Co.: New York, 1973), Chap. 4
10. van Oss, C. J., Gillman, C. F., and Good, R. J. The influence of the shape

of phagocytes on their adhesiveness. *Immunol. Commun. 1*, 627 (1972).

11. van Oss, C. J. and Mohn, J. F. Scanning electron microscopy of red cell agglutination. *Vox Sang. 19*, 432 (1970).

12. Pollack, W., Hager, H. J., Reckel, R., Toren, D. A., and Singher, H. O. A study of the forces involved in the second stage of hemagglutination. *Transfusion 5*, 158 (1965).

13. Race, R. R. An "incomplete" antibody in human serum. *Nature 153*, 771 (1944).

14. Wiener, A. S. A new test (blocking test) for Rh sensitization. *Proc. Soc. Exptl. Biol. 56*, 173 (1944).

TRIPARTITE COMPREHENSIVE COMPATIBILITY PROCEDURE

After donor blood has been selected for transfusion on the basis of the same ABO and Rh_0(D) blood groups as the patient's, pretransfusion compatibility tests with the red cells of the donor and the serum of the recipient must be performed before any transfusion can be administered. This major crossmatch is based on the premise that the recipient may possess a large pool of antibodies into which incompatible erythrocytes may be introduced, resulting in antigen-antibody unions manifested as a transfusion reaction.

To insure a maximum margin of safety, each transfusion should be preceded by a three-part compatibility procedure in which the serum of the recipient is reacted with the red cells of the donor at (1) room temperature, (2) $37°C$ in a high protein milieu, and (3) $37°C$ followed by an antiglobulin test. The room temperature test is designed to detect antibodies with in vitro temperature optima below that of body temperature but still having potential in vivo activity (anti-Le^a, anti-Le^b, anti-M, anti-N, anti-P_1, etc.). The high protein test at $37°C$ is intended to detect antibodies with in vitro optima of $37°C$ whose activity is enhanced by an increase in the protein concentration of the reaction milieu (anti-Rh, especially anti-c). The indirect antiglobulin test is carried out to detect antibodies not demonstrable by the first two direct agglutination tests (anti-Fy^a, anti-Jk^a, anti-K, etc.). It is important to appreciate that the antiglobulin test alone cannot be performed in lieu of the two direct agglutination tests. Antiglobulin reagents prepared in a single dilution, as is the case with all those available commercially, cannot be relied on to detect all orders of antibodies.

The use of enzymes in compatibility tests is contraindicated for several reasons. Not only do enzymes destroy the red cell receptors of the clinically important Fy^a (Duffy) and S (MNSs system) antigens, but one-stage enzyme tests may result in the destruction of weakly reacting antibodies in the serum of the recipient. Two-stage enzyme tests complicate the performance of the crossmatch tests unnecessarily with no practical improvement in the safety of the blood transfusion, at least when the other techniques included in a comprehensive compatibility procedure are properly designed and carried out. Enzyme techniques must never be used as the only tests in a pretransfusion compatibility procedure.

As stated in a previous exercise (Determination of ABO and Rh_0(D) Blood Groups), only approximately 35 to 40% of newborn infants possess demonstrable isoagglutinins which are all passively derived from the mother by transplacental filtration. Those present at birth regularly disappear from the infant's circulation usually within the first seven to ten days of life. It is because of this situation that in the preparation for any transfusion of an infant in the first seven to ten days of life, the maternal serum rather than the infant's own serum is routinely used in the crossmatch test. In multiple exchange transfusions of an infant suffering from hemolytic disease of the newborn, serum from the infant obtained after the first or preceding exchange should be included in these tests together with the mother's serum.

In the compatibility procedure outlined in detail here, the three phases are performed simultaneously as three separate tests each with its own control tube in which phosphate-buffered saline solution is substituted for the recipient's serum. In each tube the donor's erythrocytes are sedimented from a saline suspension by centrifugation with the supernatant solution being decanted off as completely as possible. These packed cells are then resuspended in recipient's serum, with the set of tubes for the high protein phase receiving 30% bovine serum albumin solution to raise the protein concentration to approximately 14 to 15%. The use of packed donor cells results in practically no dilution of the recipient's serum more readily permitting the detection of weak antibodies that will not withstand further dilution and still be recognized. Methods employing donor cell suspensions require microscopic examination of the reactions in an attempt to overcome the reduction in the sensitivity of the test.

This procedure, carried out as three separate tests, permits each phase to be performed under optimum conditions of incubation without extending the time required unnecessarily. In addition, each of the phases can be reexamined separately if required. These reactions should be observed for agglutination macroscopically because microscopic examination renders the test oversensitive and unnecessarily complicates the interpretation of the results. One-tube and two-tube compatibility procedures in which the tests are carried out sequentially are relatively easy to perform, but they represent a compromise in the incubation time of one or two of the phases in an attempt to keep the time required within practical limits.

Materials

1. Patient's serum, undiluted, active
2. Donor's blood, in ACD or CPD solution
3. 30% bovine serum albumin solution
4. Antihuman globulin serum (rabbit) (Coombs reagent)
5. 0.9% phosphate-buffered saline solution, pH 7.4 (PBS)
6. Pipette, capillary (Pasteur), disposable, length 5½ in.
7. Centrifuge, Sorvall Cell Washing, Model CW-1 with DA-12 Dual Angle Rotor
8. Automatic Filling Unit, Sorvall Model AF-2
9. Applicators, wood, plain
10. Tubes, culture, without rim, 10 x 75 and 12 x 75 mm

Method

1. Cut off both sealed ends of plastic integral donor tube segment and allow ACD or CPD whole blood to flow into approximately 2 ml of 0.9% phosphate-buffered saline solution (PBS) in a 12 x 75 mm tube.

Note: If donor's blood is clotted, rim gently with applicators to produce good, free-cell suspension in the serum and transfer a sufficient volume of the serum-cell suspension to 2 ml of 0.9% PBS in a 12 x 75 mm tube.

2. Centrifuge at 1200 g for 1 minute (3600 rpm Sorvall Model CW-1, DA-12 Dual Angle Rotor).
3. Decant supernatant as completely as possible.
4. Add sufficient 0.9% PBS to produce approximately 2% colorimetric suspension of cells.
5. Label six 10 x 75 mm tubes AS, A, BS, B, CS, C plus the crossmatch number (e.g., AS 5, A 5, BS 5, B 5, CS 5, C 5, etc.).
6. Place 3 drops of 2% donor's cell suspension into each tube.
7. Centrifuge at 1200 g for 1 minute.
8. Decant supernatants as completely as possible.
9. Add patient's serum as follows:

tube AS	3 drops
tube BS	2 drops
tube CS	3 drops

10. Add 0.9% PBS as follows:

tube A	3 drops
tube B	2 drops
tube C	3 drops

11. Add 1 drop of 30% bovine albumin to each of tubes BS and B.
12. Mix contents by shaking tubes gently.
13. Incubate for 15 minutes as follows:

tubes AS and A	room temperature
tubes BS and B	37°C waterbath
tubes CS and C	37°C waterbath

14. Centrifuge tubes AS, A, BS, and B at 1200 g for 1 minute.
15. Immediately reincubate tubes BS and B in the 37°C waterbath for 5 minutes.
16. Examine tubes AS, A, BS, and B macroscopically for agglutination, reading tubes BS and B directly from the 37°C waterbath.
17. Place tubes CS and C in centrifuge rotor (DA-12 Dual Angle Rotor).
18. Place the distributor manifold over the rotor knob and rotate until the 3 pins engage in the 3 holes on the rotor making certain the distributor is flush with the rotor.
19. Mount rotor by fitting it over the motor shaft and engaging the holes in the bottom plate of the rotor onto the pins of the rotating centrifuge bowl.
20. Close centrifuge cover making certain the cover latch is securely fastened.
21. Turn CW-1 centrifuge cycle selector to "Auto."
22. Turn AF-2 filling unit wash cycle selctor to "4."
23. Press signal button on AF-2 filling unit.
24. When buzzer sounds, remove rotor from centrifuge and take off distributor manifold.
25. Shake rotor gently to dislodge cell sediments.
26. Add 2 drops of antihuman globulin serum (Coombs reagent) to each tube.
27. Shake rotor gently to mix contents at once.
28. Reinsert rotor rapidly into centrifuge and close centrifuge cover.
29. Turn CW-1 centrifuge cycle selector to "Low" on left or Auto side of dial at once.
30. Turn timer to 60 seconds immediately.

Note: Centrifuge will run at 130 g for 60 seconds (1150 to 1200 rpm Sorvall Model CW-1).

31. Without delay, examine tubes macroscopically for agglutination and record the results in Protocol 4.5.

Protocol 4.5.   Tripartite Comprehensive Compatibility Procedure

Test	Tube	Crossmatch numbers		
		1	2	3
room	AS			
temperature	A			
37°C	BS			
high protein	B			
37°C	CS			
(Coombs)	C			

REFERENCES

1. Mollison, P. L. *Blood Transfusion in Clinical Medicine*, 5th ed. (Blackwell Scientific Publications, Ltd.: Oxford, 1972), pp. 202, 404.
2. Strumia, M. M., Crosby, W. H., Gibson, J. G., 2nd, Greenwalt, T. J., and Krevans, J. R., Eds., *General Principles of Blood Transfusion* (J. B. Lippincott Co.: Philadelphia, 1963). Published originally in *Transfusion 3*, 303 (1963).

TESTS FOR THE DETECTION OF ANTIBODY SENSITIZATION OF ERYTHROCYTES

The year following their introduction of a new procedure for demonstrating incomplete anti-Rh antibodies in maternal sera--the indirect antiglobulin test or indirect Coombs test--Coombs, Mourant, and Race reported their studies on the application of this technique for the detection of in vivo antibody sensitization of the erythrocytes of babies with hemolytic disease of the newborn. The results clearly showed that this procedure, now referred to as the direct antiglobulin test or direct Coombs test, provided a reliable means for rapid determination of the presence of antibody-coated red cells. This serologic information alerts the physician to the possibility of the development of hemolytic disease of the newborn in the immediate neonatal period, especially if there were no clinically overt signs and symptoms of this disease at birth.

In their original paper, one very interesting case was noted in which the newborn infant showed a positive direct antiglobulin test although the mother was Rh_0(D) positive as well as the father and the affected infant, all three belonging to the Rh group R_1 r. Using the indirect antiglobulin method, the maternal serum was found to be negative against cells representing all the known Rh antigens, sensitizing strongly only the father's red cells. This later was proved to be the discovery of a "new" blood group antigen, K antigen, the first one found in the Kell system. This illustrates the importance of the development of a new serologic technique in demonstrating isoantibodies previously not detectable by standard methods.

Gurevitch, Polishuk, and Hermoni in 1947 examined the serum enhancement effect of umbilical cord sera and the sera of children from one to eighteen months of age in comparison with normal adult sera on incomplete anti-Rh and immune anti-A sera. They found that umbilical cord sera and the sera of infants of up to six months of age were devoid of enhancing properties.

The same year Witebsky, Rubin, and Blum published their findings on the capacity of prenatal and postnatal sera to activate incomplete anti-Rh antibodies to produce direct agglutination. They found that when cord sera of full-term newborn infants were compared with normal adult sera, the results were dependent on the potency of the anti-Rh sera being examined. In all instances the average, normal cord serum proved to be of weaker potency than the average normal adult serum. A striking difference was demonstrated between the cord sera of premature infants and of those born at term when incomplete anti-Rh sera of high titer were used. In their opinion, this activating power of serum diluent is dependent on a maturation principle subject to considerable individual variation.

As a consequence of these studies Witebsky, Rubin, Engasser, and Blum developed a simple technique for the demonstration of antibody-sensitization of the red cells of infants with hemolytic disease of the newborn. When packed erythrocytes prepared from cord blood specimens, from which as much of the serum had been removed as possible by centrifugation, were suspended in undiluted, normal, adult, human group AB serum (or other ABO compatible serum) on a slide, spontaneous agglutination of the antibody-coated cells occurred. They concluded that the cord serum was similar to saline solution in its inability to effect agglutination of erythrocytes sensitized in vivo by incomplete anti-Rh antibodies. Later Witebsky augmented this test by adding a diluent composed of equal parts of undiluted, adult, human group AB serum (or other ABO compatible serum) and 30% bovine serum albumin solution in addition to the serum itself. He showed that the serum+albumin mixture was the superior diluent for detecting sensitization of the infant's red cells in Rh hemolytic disease of the newborn, a not surprising finding since it paralleled the experience with this diluent in determining the titer of incomplete anti-Rh antibodies in maternal sera.

This slide sensitization test has proved to be invaluable in detecting anti-body-coating of infants' erythrocytes in cases of ABO hemolytic desease of the newborn. When the ABO blood group system is involved in isoimmunization of pregnancy, the direct antiglobulin test (direct Coombs test) that is invariably positive in 100% of cases of Rh hemolytic disease of the newborn has proved to be inadequate in the hands of many investigators. In our own experience with the most optimum antihuman globulin sera (rabbit), positive results have been obtained in no more than 40% of cases. In contrast, 80% have been positive in the Witebsky slide sensitization test.

Experience has confirmed the importance of using both diluents in the test, the undiluted, adult serum and the serum+albumin mixture. In the same investigation in which he proved the value of this test in ABO hemolytic disease of the newborn, Witebsky pointed out that the serum+albumin diluent, by far the more superior in activating incomplete anti-D antibodies in maternal sera, was definitely inferior to undiluted, adult sera in activating immune anti-A antibodies in maternal serum in his partial neutralization procedure. A similar experience prevails with the Witebsky slide sensitization test in that positive results are obtained with the infants' cells sensitized by immune anti-A anti-bodies in this serum diluent in contrast to the serum+albumin mixture that yields the most positive reactions in Rh cases. In fact, it is often possible to predict ABO versus Rh hemolytic disease of the newborn by a careful observation of the agglutination reaction patterns occurring in these two diluents in the slide sensitization test.

In the same year that the application of the antiglobulin technique in the serologic detection of antibody-sensitization of erythrocytes in Rh hemolytic disease of the newborn was described, Boorman, Dodd, and Loutit reported their findings with this procedure in examining erythrocytes from patients with congenital and acquired hemolytic anemia. Positive direct antiglobulin tests were obtained in all their cases diagnosed as acquired hemolytic anemia (acquired acholuric jaundice) on the basis of clinical, hematologic, and biochemical data in contrast to negative results in every case believed to be congenital hemolytic anemia (congenital acholuric jaundice). This cardinal observation was the first step in establishing unequivocally the immunologic evidence for autoantibody formation in acquired hemolytic anemia. Today it is the most important test in confirming serologically the clinical diagnosis of autoimmune hemolytic anemia.

The Witebsky slide sensitization test is also useful in this disease. Both types of serologic patterns have been observed in adults with autoimmune hemolytic anemia analogous to the findings in serum and serum+albumin diluents with ABO and Rh hemolytic disease of the newborn, respectively.

Again, Witebsky found that on occasion this test gave positive results when the direct antiglobulin test was negative in examining the erythrocytes from persons suspected of having autoimmune hemolytic anemia.

Slide Serum and Serum+Albumin Sensitization Test (Witebsky)

Materials

1. Patient's blood, clotted, cord or peripheral
2. Control blood, clotted, peripheral, normal, adult
3. Human serum, group AB, undiluted, normal, native, adult
4. Human serum+bovine albumin mixture of equal parts group AB, undiluted, normal, native, adult, human serum and 30% bovine serum albumin
5. 0.9% phosphate-buffered saline solution, pH 7.4 (PBS)
6. Viewing box, light-heat
7. Slide, 6 x 3 in., with 15 permanently marked ceramic ovals
8. Timer, interval
9. Pipette, capillary (Pasteur), disposable, length 5½ in.
10. Applicators, wood, plain
11. Tubes, centrifuge, conical, polycarbonate, capacity 15 ml
12. Tubes, culture, without rim, 12 x 100 mm

Method

1. With separate applicators, rim each clot gently to produce heavy, free-cell suspensions in the sera.
2. Decant the serum-cell suspensions into properly prelabeled, conical centrifuge tubes.
3. Centrifuge at 1345 g for 5 minutes (3600 rpm Sorvall Model CW-1, CP12-3 General Purpose Angle Rotor) or at 733 g for 10 minutes (2000 rpm Sorvall Model GLC-1, HL-4 Horizontal Rotor with no. 548 Omni-Carrier and no. 565 Stainless Steel Insert, 6-place).
4. Remove the supernatant serum from each as completely as possible with separate Pasteur pipettes and place into prelabeled 12 x 100 mm tubes.
5. Using separate Pasteur pipettes, place 2 drops of each of the following diluents in each of 2 ovals in the horizontal rows according to the protocol as follows:

row a	human group AB serum
row b	human serum+bovine albumin mixture
row c	patient's serum
row d	0.9% PBS

6. Using separate Pasteur pipettes, add 1 drop of packed red cells to each oval in the vertical rows according to the protocol as follows:

    row 1   control cells
    row 2   patient's cells

7. Mix contents of ovals thoroughly, using separate applicators for each.
8. Switch on light in viewing box and set timer for 10 minutes.
9. Examine the mixture for 10 minutes while constantly rotating the viewing box to mix gently the contents of the ovals.

Note: *It is advisable to switch off the light in the viewing box periodically to prevent the slide from getting too warm, thereby causing the blood mixtures to dry.*

10. After 10 minutes of constant rotation and observation, record in Protocol 4.6 the final agglutination results obtained.

Tube Direct Antiglobulin Sensitization Test (Coombs)

Materials

1. Patient's blood, clotted, cord or peripheral
2. Control blood, clotted, peripheral, normal, adult
3. Antihuman globulin serum (rabbit) (Coombs reagent)
4. 0.9% phosphate-buffered saline solution, pH 7.4 (PBS), cold (stored at 4°C)
5. Centrifuge, Sorvall Cell Washing, Model CW-1 with DA-12 Dual Angle Rotor
6. Automatic Filling Unit, Sorvall Model AF-2
7. Applicators, wood, plain
8. Tubes, culture, without rim, 10 x 75 mm

Method

1. Rim each clot with separate applicators until the dislodged red cells form approximately 3% colorimetric suspensions in the sera.
2. Place 2 drops of each 3% cell suspension into prelabeled 10 x 75 mm tubes.
3. Place tubes in centrifuge rotor (DA-12 Dual Angle Rotor).
4. Place the distributor manifold over the rotor knob and rotate until the 3 pins engage in the 3 holes on the rotor making certain the distributor is flush with the rotor.

5. Mount rotor by fitting it over the motor shaft and engaging the holes in the bottom plate of the rotor onto the pins of the rotating centrifuge bowl.
6. Close centrifuge cover making certain the cover latch is securely fastened.
7. Turn CW-1 centrifuge cycle selector to "Auto."
8. Turn AF-2 filling unit wash cycle selector to "4."
9. Press signal button on AF-2 filling unit.
10. When buzzer sounds, remove rotor from centrifuge and take off distributor manifold.
11. Shake rotor gently to dislodge cell sediments.
12. Add 2 drops of antihuman globulin serum (Coombs reagent) to each tube.
13. Shake rotor gently to mix contents at once.
14. Reinsert rotor rapidly into centrifuge and close centrifuge cover.
15. Turn CW-1 centrifuge cycle selector to "Low" on left or Auto side of dial at once.
16. Turn timer to 60 seconds immediately.

Note: *Centrifuge will run at 130 g for 60 seconds (1150-1200 rpm Sorvall Model CW-1).*

17. Without delay, examine each tube macroscopically for agglutination and record the results in Protocol 4.7.

Note: *The control tube containing the normal, adult cells should be negative.*

Protocol 4.6.   Slide Serum and Serum+Albumin Sensitization Test (Witebsky)

		1 drop packed, unwashed red cells		
		Control 1	Patient no. 1 2	Patient no. 2 3
(a)	Human serum 2 drops			
(b)	Human serum + bovine albumin mixture 2 drops			
(c)	Patient's serum 2 drops			
(d)	Saline 2 drops			

Protocol 4.7.   Tube Direct Antiglobulin Sensitization Test (Coombs)

	2 drops 3% cell suspension		
	Control	Patient no. 1	Patient no. 2
	1	2	3

Antiglobulin serum   2 drops

Each new lot of antihuman globulin serum that is used should be tested with a positive control. If it is to be stored for any length of time at 4°C, it should also be tested at least once a month in order to detect any undesirable decrease in its antibody content. It is also important to include cells sensitized with antibody as a positive control whenever antiglobulin tests are performed. Such sensitized cells can be obtained from commercial sources. A positive control can also be prepared in the following manner:

1.   Select a fresh, normal, human adult blood of group O which is strongly Rh_0(D) positive in the routine Rh grouping.
2.   Wash the cells three times with copious volumes of cold PBS.
3.   Prepare a 3% suspension of the washed cells in PBS.
4.   Place 2 drops of this cell suspension in a 10 x 75 mm tube.
5.   Add 2 drops of incomplete (albumin) anti-D serum (Slide Test or Modified Tube Test Anti-D serum).
6.   Mix the contents of the tube thoroughly.
7.   Incubate for 30 minutes in a 37°C waterbath.
8.   After the incubation period, proceed from step 3 of the Tube Direct Antiglobulin Sensitization Test (Coombs) procedure.
9.   If the control was prepared properly and if the antiglobulin reagent is really potent, agglutination will be readily observed in this tube.

REFERENCES

1.   Boorman, K. E., Dodd, B. E., and Loutit, J. F. Haemolytic icterus (acholuric jaundice) congenital and acquired. *Lancet i*, 812 (1946).
2.   Coombs, R. R. A., Mourant, A. E., and Race, R. R. A new test for the detection of weak and "incomplete" Rh agglutinins. *Brit. J. Exptl. Path.* 26, 255 (1945).

3. —————————. In-vivo isosensitisation of red cells in babies with haemolytic disease. *Lancet i*, 264 (1946).
4. Gurevitch, J., Polishuk, Z., and Hermoni, D. The role of a presumed serum protein in the pathogenesis of erythroblastosis fetalis. *Amer. J. Clin. Path.* *17*, 465 (1947).
5. Witebsky, E. The immunology of acquired hemolytic anemia: diagnostic and therapeutic consideration. *Proc. 4th Congr. Int. Soc. Hemat.*, Mar del Plata 1952 (Grune & Stratton: New York, 1954), p. 284.
6. Witebsky, E., Rubin, M. I., and Blum, L. Studies in erythroblastosis fetalis. I. Activation of the incomplete Rh antibody by the blood serum of full-term and premature newborn infants. *J. Lab. Clin. Med. 32*, 1330 (1947).
7. Witebsky, E., Rubin, M. I., Engasser, L. M., and Blum, L. Studies in erythroblastosis fetalis. II. Investigations on the detection of sensitization of the red blood cells of newborn infants with erythroblastosis fetalis. *J. Lab. Clin. Med. 32*, 1339 (1947).

Chapter 5

PROCEDURES USING LABELED ANTIBODIES OR ANTIGENS

P. Bigazzi   J. Puleo
K. Wicher   G. Andres
E. Gorzynski   S. Gutcho
R. Zeschke

IMMUNOFLUORESCENCE

Immunofluorescence (IF) is a technique that allows the localization of antigens at the cellular level using their corresponding antibodies labeled with a fluorescent dye so that they become visible under the fluorescent microscope. Applying the same principle, antibodies can be localized at the cellular level, using their corresponding antigen labeled with a fluorescent compound. IF has become increasingly useful both for research and diagnosis in the fields of immunology and microbiology. Using this procedure, unknown antigens have been identified and the presence of known antigens in tissues and microorganisms has been verified, as well as the localization of antigen-antibody complexes and complement in some tissues. The presence of circulating antibodies against tissue, microbial or viral antigens has been determined in human or animal sera.

Several variations of the IF technique have been successfully utilized, but those most commonly used for diagnostic purposes are the following:

(1) Direct method, in which fluorescein-labeled antibody is applied to a preparation containing the corresponding antigen. With the direct method, immunoglobulins and complement presumably associated with antigen-antibody complexes can be detected in kidney or skin biopsies. Kidney biopsies of patients with glomerulonephritis or certain other kidney diseases can be examined for IgG, IgA, IgM, and complement. Skin biopsies of patients with bullous diseases that are examined by the same method reveal a number of staining patterns that are of differential diagnostic value.

(2) Indirect method, in which antigen is treated with its corresponding unlabeled antibody; the resulting antigen-antibody complex is treated with a fluorescein-labeled antibody to the immunoglobulin of the animal species that

107

provided the unlabeled antibody used in the first step. Antibodies to antigens in nuclei, skin, stomach, striated or smooth muscle, thyroid, adrenals, ovary, testis, and so on, have been detected by the indirect method in sera of patients with a variety of autoimmune diseases.

As already mentioned, IF is also useful in the diagnosis of bacterial, parasitic, and viral infections: the fluorescent treponemal antibody absorption test is at present considered the most specific test in the serodiagnosis of syphilis, and IF procedures are employed in the diagnosis of toxoplasmosis, trachoma, cytomegalovirus infections, and animal rabies. However, the number of instances in which this technique is of practical diagnostic value in the field of microbiology is rather limited, mainly because of the problem of the specificity of the reagents. The preparation of highly specific conjugates in most cases is difficult owing to the presence of cross-reactive antigens and a large number of serotypes.

For a detailed discussion on the basic principles and the latest developments in fluorescence microscopy, filters, condensers, preparation of conjugates and so on, reference books completely devoted to this subject should be consulted (4-5, 7-8). In the following pages only a brief outline will be given on some of the reagents employed in diagnostic IF methods.

Antigens

Tissue sections, tissue-culture monolayers, imprint smears from various organs, smears of cells, exudates or cultures of microorganisms can be used as sources of antigens. Tissues are snap-frozen in liquid nitrogen (or with dry ice if no liquid nitrogen is available) and kept in dry ice until they are used, which in most cases should be as soon as possible. In some instances they may be stored at −70°C for long periods of time, which vary with the antigen involved. Thyroid microsomal antigens retain their reactivity at about −20°C for two to three weeks, while thyroglobulin may last for several months. Most viral antigens are quite stable and can be stored at −70°C for several weeks.

Tissue sections are cut in a cryostat at 4μ (sections should not be thicker than that to avoid nonspecific staining) and air-dried. Tissue-culture monolayers can be grown on coverslips in Leighton tubes, and smears can be prepared as for normal staining techniques.

The substrate material has to be prepared and attached to the slide so as to preserve as much as possible both its histological structure and its immunological reactivity. Since the use of fixatives can affect the latter, it would be desirable not to fix the substrate. This can actually be done with sections of some tissues, while for some other tissues, a short fixation in acetone, ethanol, or methanol may be helpful. Infectious materials should be fixed to inactivate the bacteria or the viruses under examination, while at the same time preserving their antigenicity as well as the cellular structure of infected tissues or cell monolayers. For most viruses the best fixative is acetone, used at room temperature or at 4°C or at −20°C for periods of time ranging from 30 seconds to 2-4 hours.

Antisera

Hemolysis should be prevented, since degradation of immunoglobulin can be caused by enzyme action. Bacterial contamination should also be avoided as it interferes both with the stability of antibodies in the serum and the reading of the tests under the fluorescent microscope. Blood should be collected and serum should be separated with sterile glassware. Sera may be filtered through micropore filters, divided into small aliquots, frozen, and kept at −20°C or lower. Repeated freezing and thawing causes a rapid loss of antibody activity. Sera should be diluted in phosphate-buffered saline before use, since undiluted sera cause a high degree of nonspecific staining.

Control sera should be included in every experiment, i.e. known positive sera at various dilutions and sera that are expected to be negative. When using patients' sera, one should add as negative controls sera from patients with a variety of diseases, especially those affecting the organ under study and those with an increase in serum γ globulins.

Antisera to γ Globulins, Conjugated with
Fluorescein Isothiocyanate (FITC-Conjugates)

The preparation and standardization of FITC-conjugates are rather complex; for details, recent publications on this subject should be consulted (1-3, 6). In practice, however, laboratories using IF procedures for diagnostic purposes should be able to use commercially available FITC-conjugates, just as other commercial reagents are employed for various diagnostic procedures. The information provided by the manufacturers should include characterization by immunoelectrophoresis; antibody content; protein content; fluorescein-to-protein, antibody-to-fluorescein, and antibody-to-protein ratios; and, of course, the dilution range at which the conjugate itself should be used for the most common diagnostic tests.

If a correlation of results obtained in different diagnostic laboratories is desired, a standard conjugate from a reference standard center might be used alongside the commercial conjugate, to obtain an estimation of potency as is already done for many biological products. Changing the lot of conjugate or the test in which the conjugate is used (e.g., determination of thyroid antibodies instead of the FTA test) would require another comparison with the standard conjugate.

Phosphate-Buffered Saline (PBS), pH 7.2

Sera and conjugates are diluted with PBS at pH 7.2 (p. 201). It has been observed that the fluorescence intensity of FITC-conjugates changes with pH and reaches a maximum at pH 8.0, and therefore pH values higher than the conventional pH 7.2 have been suggested as optimal by some investigators. It has also been observed that nonspecific staining decreases at pH 8.5. Before such a change is universally accepted, more accurate trials are needed.

Mounting Fluid

The most commonly used is a mixture of nine parts glycerol (analytical reagent grade) and one part PBS. As already stated for PBS, changes in pH of mounting fluid have been suggested, since high pH increases the intensity of staining. Other mounting fluids are commercially available.

REFERENCES

1. Beutner, E. H., Ed. Defined immunofluorescence staining. *Ann. N. Y. Acad. Sci. 177*, 1 (1971).
2. Beutner, E. H., Ed. *Immunofluorescence* (in preparation).
3. Beutner, E. H., Chorzelski, T. P., and Jordan, R. E., Eds. *Autosensitization in Pemphigus and Bullous Pemphigoid*, (Thomas: Springfield, Ill. 1970).
4. Beutner, E. H. and Nisengard, R., Eds. *Manual for Immunofluorescence in Clinical Immunopathology* Department of Microbiology, SUNY at Buffalo, School of Medicine, Buffalo (1971).
5. Goldman, M., Ed. *Fluorescent Antibody Methods* (Academic: New York, 1968).
6. Holborow, E. J., Ed. *Standardization in Immunofluorescence* (Blackwell: Oxford, 1970).
7. Kawamura, A., Jr., Ed. *Fluorescent Antibody Techniques and Their Applications* (U. of Tokyo and University Park: Tokyo and Baltimore, 1969).
8. Nairn, R. C., Ed. *Fluorescent Protein Tracing* (William and Wilkins: Baltimore, 1969).

Direct IF Staining

Immunoglobulins Fixed to Tissues. The immunofluorescent technique is of great value in the diagnosis of renal disease. Sections of kidney biopsies from patients with different renal diseases are stained by fluorescein-conjugated antisera to human γ globulins and complement, and different patterns of staining may be observed.

In patients with an immune complex glomerulonephritis (lupus nephritis, poststreptococcal, malarial, membranous and membranous proliferative glomerulonephritis), granular or broad irregular deposits of immunoglobulins can be observed along the glomerular basement membrane. In patients with an antiglomerular basement membrane antibody disease (glomerulonephritis associated with Goodpasture's syndrome, rapidly progressive glomerulonephritis), a continuous linear staining for IgG and complement can be observed along the glomerular basement membrane. The immunofluorescent method is particularly useful in the differential diagnosis between membranous glomerulonephritis (characterized by immune complexes) and lipoid nephrosis (no deposits of immunoglobulins) and between poststreptococcal glomerulonephritis (scanty granular deposits) and membranous proliferative glomerulonephritis (abundant deposits of complement and IgG).

Materials

1.   Cryostat sections of biopsy of human kidney (4μ, unfixed, air-dried)
2.   FITC-conjugate to human γ globulins
3.   Phosphate-buffered saline (PBS), pH 7.2 (p. 205)
4.   Mounting fluid (p. 110)

Method

1.   Rinse and wash the sections with PBS for 10 minutes.
2.   Cover the preparation with appropriately diluted FITC-conjugate and incubate for 30-60 minutes at room temperature. (As a control, some sections should be treated with a conjugate to a different antigen. Blocking tests and treatment of normal kidney sections with conjugate to human γ globulins can also be used.)
3.   Rinse and wash with PBS for 30 minutes.
4.   Dry carefully the area around the section, but do not allow the preparations to dry. Add one drop of mounting fluid on the slide, cover with coverslip, and read under an ultraviolet microscope.

REFERENCE

1.   McCluskey, R. T. The value of immunofluorescence in the study of human renal disease. *J. Exptl. Med.* *134*, 242S (1971).

Identification of Group A Streptococci. Streptococci account for more infectious diseases than all other organisms combined. The group A streptococci play the most important part in streptococcal infections, and speedy isolation and identification is of clinical importance.

After the beta hemolytic, bacitracin-sensitive streptococcus is isolated, accurate identification can be done by means of capillary precipitin test or fluorescent antibody technique (IF). Assuming that a proper conjugate is available (specific antiserum to streptococcus, group A, conjugated with fluorescent isothiocyanate), the IF test is preferred because of the simplicity and reproducibility.

Materials

1.   Streptococci cultured on blood agar or on Streptosel, a fluid medium. An 18-hour culture is suspended in PBS and spread on a microscope slide, or when Streptosel is used, the bacterial suspension is applied directly on the slide. Smears are fixed in 95% alcohol and air-dried.
2.   FITC-conjugated rabbit antiserum containing group-specific antibodies
3.   Phosphate-buffered saline (PBS), pH 7.4 (p. 205)
4.   Mounting fluid (p. 110)

Method

1.   Apply the appropriately diluted FITC-conjugated antiserum and incubate at room temperature for 30 minutes.
2.   Wash in PBS for 10 minutes and rinse with distilled water.
3.   Add a drop of mounting fluid on the slide, cover with a coverslip, and examine under an ultraviolet microscope.

REFERENCES

1.   Cherry, W. B. and Moody, M. D. Fluorescent antibody techniques in diagnostic bacteriology. *Bact. Rev. 29*, 222 (1965).
2.   Moody, M. D., Ellis, E. C., and Updyke, E. L. Staining bacterial smears with fluorescent antibody. IV. Grouping streptococci with fluorescent antibody. *J. Bacteriol. 75*, 553 (1958).

Demonstration of Rabies Virus Antigen. The laboratory diagnosis of animal rabies can be performed by several methods, but at present the most commonly used is the direct IF technique (fluorescent rabies antibody or FRA test). The

FRA test gives a prompt result, is positive at almost any stage of the disease, and can demonstrate rabies virus antigen even when infectivity studies by mouse inoculation are negative because of inactivation of the virus by heat or antibodies or in the case of strains with low pathogenicity. Positive results by the FRA test have been reported in 99.4% of cases, while the mouse inoculation test was positive in 98.3% and the microscopic examination for Negri bodies was positive in 65.8%.

Materials

1. Smears of CNS tissue (hippocampus, cerebellum, medulla, cerebrum, brain stem) or salivary gland tissue. As positive controls smears from entire brains of young mice inoculated intracerebrally with rabies virus are used, while the inhibition test is used to check specificity of strain. Some normal mouse brains produce autofluorescence. The sections are air-dried, then the slides are placed in a slide container, covered with cold acetone, left for two to four hours in a freezer at between −15 and −20°C, then removed from the acetone, and air-dried. Slides should be handled and disposed of as contaminated material.
2. Antirabies serum conjugated with fluorescein isothiocyanate. This conjugate is prepared by fractionating with ammonium sulfate hyperimmune hamster antirabies serum and labeling the γ globulins with FITC. The conjugate is then run through a Sephadex G-50 column and lyophilized.
3. Phosphate-buffered saline (PBS), pH 7.4 (p. 205)
4. Mounting fluid (p. 110)

Method

1. Place two drops of diluted conjugate on the smears.
2. Incubate at 37°C in a humidified chamber for 30 minutes.
3. Remove slides from incubator and wash with PBS and distilled water.
4. Dry, add one drop of mounting fluid, cover with a coverslip, and examine under a fluorescence microscope. Smears positive for rabies antigen will contain brilliant apple-green fluorescent structures of varying size, ranging from tiny bodies called viral sand, or dust, to the larger classical Negri bodies.

REFERENCE

1. Lennette, W. H. and Schmidt, N. J., Eds. *Diagnostic Procedures for Viral and Rickettsial Diseases* (American Public Health Assoc., New York, 1969).

Indirect IF Staining

Antinuclear Antibodies (ANA). The detection of ANA is extremely helpful in the diagnosis of systemic lupus erythematosus (SLE), since practically all patients with active untreated SLE have circulating antibodies to nuclear antigens. ANA are also present with a lower incidence in other diseases, such as rheumatoid arthritis, scleroderma, and dermatomyositis. Cryostat sections of mouse liver are most commonly used for the detection of circulating ANA, but various tissues from various animals can also be employed, since these antibodies do not exhibit species or organ specificity. The binding of antibodies to nuclear antigens can be detected by FITC-conjugates to human IgG, IgM, and IgA. Different patterns of staining are observed, that is, "diffuse" or "homogeneous," "peripheral," "speckled," and "nucleolar" staining.

Materials

1. Cryostat sections of mouse liver (4μ, unfixed)
2. Patient's serum and control sera
3. Rabbit or goat antiserum to human γ globulins, FITC-conjugated
4. Phosphate-buffered saline (PBS) pH 7.2
5. Mounting fluid

Method

1. Cover tissue sections with different dilutions of serum to be tested. Some sections should be covered with control sera. A serum known to contain ANA should be used as a positive control, and a serum without ANA should be the negative control. Some sections should be treated with PBS as a control of nonspecific staining of the conjugate.
2. Incubate sections for 30 minutes at room temperature in a humid chamber.
3. Rinse and wash sections with gentle stirring in PBS for 30-45 minutes.
4. Cover sections with appropriately diluted FITC-conjugate and incubate for 30 minutes.
5. Rinse and wash with PBS for 30-45 minutes.
6. Mount in buffered glycerine and read under UV microscope.

REFERENCES

1. Barnett, E. V. Substrates for antinuclear factors. In: Holborow, E. J., Ed. *Standardization in Immunofluorescence* (Blackwell: Oxford, 1970) p. 75.

2. Beck, J. S. Antinuclear antibodies: Methods of detection and significance. *Mayo Clinic Proc.* **44**, 600 (1969).
3. Bickel, Y. B., Barnett, E. V., and Pearson, C. M. Immunofluorescent patterns and specificity of human antinuclear antibodies. *Clin. Exptl. Immunol.* **3**, 641 (1968).
4. Dorsch, C. A., et al. Significance of nuclear immunofluorescent patterns. *Ann. Pheum. Dis.* **28**, 313 (1969).
5. Ritchie, R. F. Antinucleolar antibodies. *New Eng. J. Med.* **282**, 1174 (1970).

Fluorescent Treponemal Antibody Absorption (FTA-ABS) Test. Sera from patients with syphilis when tested by the indirect IF technique on smears of treponemata give a positive reaction characterized by apple-green staining of the spirochetes (fluorescent treponemal antibody, or FTA, test). Since common or group-specific antigens are shared by both pathogenic and nonpathogenic treponemata, this is a major cause of cross-reactivity of the FTA test, which is performed with patients' sera at low dilutions. To obviate this disadvantage, the fluorescent treponemal antibody absorption (FTA-ABS) test was developed, based on the absorption of common or cross-reactivity treponemal antibodies by diluting patients' sera with an extract of nonpathogenic Reiter treponemas ("Sorbent").

Materials

1. *Treponema pallidum* (pathogenic Nichols strain), lyophilized antigen
2. Anti-human-γ-globulin conjugated with FITC, lyophilized (FITC-conjugate or FTA test reagent)
3. Phosphate-buffered saline (PBS), pH 7.2
4. PBS containing 2.0% Tween 80 (PBS-T80)
5. FTA-ABS test sorbent
6. Reactive serum (TPS) control
7. Normal serum (NS) control
8. Mounting fluid (p. 110)
9. Acetone

Method

1. Heat inactivate (30 minutes in waterbath at 56°C) all test and control serum specimens.
2. Add 5.0 ml sterile, distilled water to a vial of conjugate; distribute in 0.5-1.0-ml aliquots and freeze until needed. Prior to use, this restored

conjugate must be further diluted with PBS-T80. The volume of PBS-T80 to be employed is obtained by testing with standard control sera to determine the highest dilution of conjugate giving maximum fluorescence with TPS. Final dilutions of conjugated globulin may range from 1:5 to 1:320.

3. Add 1 ml of sterile distilled water to a vial of lyophilized *T. pallidum* antigen; then deposit approximately 0.005 ml *T. pallidum* suspension in each of two circles etched onto a quantity of microslides.

4. Allow 15 minutes for thorough drying; then fix in acetone at room temperature for 10 minutes.

5. Decant acetone; and air-dry the slides. Slides may be prepared in advance and stored up to 30 days at $-20°C$ after fixation in acetone.

6. Add 0.05 ml of patient's serum (diluted 1:5 in FTA-ABS test sorbent) on a test slide. Similarly, add 0.05 ml of appropriately diluted TPS and NS to control slides.

7. Incubate test and control slides at $37°C$ for 30 minutes in a moist atmosphere to prevent evaporation.

8. Rinse slides with PBS and wash them in two changes of PBS for a total of 10 minutes, followed by a brief rinse in distilled water.

9. Blot slides gently with filter paper to remove water drops.

10. Add 0.06 ml of diluted FTA test reagent (for method of diluting, see step 2 above). Spread conjugate to cover the smears completely. Incubate at $37°C$ for 30 minutes as described in step 4.

11. Rinse, wash, and blot dry as in step 5.

12. Add a small drop of mounting fluid to each smear and apply cover glass.

13. Examine with fluorescent microscope, using a high-dry (45X magnification) objective. In the absence of fluorescence, confirm the presence of *T. pallidum* under dark-field microscopy.

REFERENCES

1. Cherry, W. B., Goldman, M., Carski, T. R., and Moody, M. D. *Fluorescent Antibody Techniques in the Diagnosis of Communicable Diseases.* U. S. Public Health Service. Pub. 729 (Washington, D. C., 1960).

2. Deacon, W. E., Falcone, V. H., and Harris, A. A fluorescent test for treponemal antibodies. *Proc. Soc. Exptl. Biol. Med. 96*, 477 (1957).

3. Deacon, W. E. and Hunter, E. F. Treponemal antigens as related to identification and syphilis serology. *Proc. Soc. Exptl. Biol. Med. 110*, 352 (1962).

4. Hunter, E. F., Deacon, W. E., and Meyer, P. E. An improved FTA test for syphilis: The absorption procedure (FTA-ABS). *Pub. Health Rep. 79*, 410

(1964).

5.   Hunter, E. F. Characteristics of patient sera, conjugates, and antigens used in FTA-ABS tests. *Ann. N. Y. Acad. Sci. 177*, 48 (1971).

IF Test for Toxoplasmosis. Toxoplasmosis is a congenital or acquired infection caused by *Toxoplasma gondii*, an ubiquitous, parasitic protozoan. While the acute form of the disease is not common, serological surveys indicate that infection is common. It seems likely that in most cases the infection is asymptomatic, the manifestations (fever, lymphadenopathy, myalgia) are not severe enough for the individual to seek medical care or that the possibility of toxoplasmosis is not considered by the physician. In those instances of acute infection, meningoencephalitis, pneumonitis, myocarditis, typhus-like exanthema, conjunctivitis, severe myalgia, and arthralgia are most often seen. Chorioretinitis appears to be most often associated with congenital toxoplasmosis and may be recurrent.

Acute toxoplasmosis has been associated with leukocyte transfusion, radiation therapy, chemotherapy and steroid therapy for malignancies, and immunosuppression therapy for transplantation. In those instances where the symptoms suggest infection with toxoplasma, the indirect IF test on smears of *T. gondii* has proven to be in agreement with the older Sabin-Feldman dye test, but unlike the dye test, it does not require live organisms and is therefore easier and safer to perform.

Materials

1.   Antigen. Antigen slides are prepared from formalin killed *T. gondii* organisms harvested from infected mouse peritoneal fluid or infected tissue culture. After washing the organisms, a sufficiently dense suspension is prepared to assure 15-30 organisms per high-dry field when smeared on a slide. After thorough air-drying, the slides are packaged and stored frozen ($-20°C$). The antigen slides may be removed from the freezer and used immediately without further treatment.
2.   Patient's serum, control sera
3.   FITC-conjugate. The fluorescein conjugated anti-human-γ-globulin should be reconstituted in 1:500 (0.2%) Evans blue in PBS to the proper volume. This should be made fresh for each determination and not stored.
4.   Phosphate-buffered saline solution (PBS), pH 7.2 (p. 205)
5.   Buffered glycerol (p. 198)

Method

1.   Using PBS, prepare serial fourfold dilutions of the serum to be tested.

Dilutions may be started at 1:16, since this is the lowest dilution that should be tested. Fourfold dilutions of sera are a minimal requirement when making comparisons on a test-to-test basis, but two-fold dilutions will give more information when comparisons of sera are to be made in the same test. The following controls should be used each time the test is performed: (a) PBS, (b)negative serum, and (c) positive human serum of known titer. The positive serum is tested at four dilutions: one below, two above, and one at the known titer of the serum. For example, if the control serum has a titer of 1024, using a fourfold dilution scheme, it should be tested at dilutions of 1:256, 1:1024, 1:4096, 1:16,384. The negative control serum should be tested at 1:64 only. When larger numbers of sera are to be tested, it is recommended that they be screened at 1:16 and 1:64 dilutions. If a serum is positive at 1:64, it should be retested at higher dilutions to determine its titer.

2. Remove antigen slides from freezer and wash in a light stream of distilled water.
3. Blot dry (facial tissue is satisfactory). Place the slides in a humid chamber and cover each smear with a different serum dilution.
4. Incubate at 37°C for 30 minutes.
5. Rinse off serum dilutions with a light stream of distilled water.
6. Immerse the slides in a staining dish containing PBS and agitate on a mechanical rotator at 10-20 rpm for 15 minutes (speed of rotation is not critical).
7. Blot the smears dry and replace the slides in a humid chamber.
8. Cover the smears with the optimal dilution of FITC-conjugate and incubate at 37°C for 30 minutes.
9. Repeat washings as previously described with a final distilled-water rinse.
10. Blot dry. Place a small drop of buffered glycerol on the smear and superimpose a coverslip.
11. Examine with a high-dry objective of a fluorescence microscope. The reaction is negative when the organisms fluoresce reddish-purple (due to Evans blue) with no yellow-green fluorescence around their periphery; it is also considered negative when only the anterior end of the organisms fluoresces bright yellow-green with no extension of yellow-green around the posterior end. This "polar staining" will occur at lower dilutions and usually disappears at a serum dilution between 1:16 and 1:64. The reaction is positive when yellow-green fluorescence extends around the entire periphery of the organism. This reaction may be intense enough (in lower dilutions of strong positive sera) to mask all internal red counterstain. In higher dilutions, the peripheral staining will become a thin peripheral halo around an internal red fluorescence. The titer of the serum is given by the

highest dilution at which more than half of the organisms exhibit the yellow-green fluorescence around their entire periphery. With fourfold dilutions, the end point usually has a sharp cutoff. Tests should always be performed on different serum samples from the same patient, because a single titer is never significant and only a changing titer gives meaningful information. Titers between 16 and 64 usually reflect only some past exposure or may indicate an early stage of the disease. Titers to 256 usually indicate relatively recent exposure or present involvement; the clinician should be alerted of this possibility. Titers of 1024 or more are very significant, and the clinician should be advised to consider toxoplasmosis and attempt to document the disease further.

REFERENCES

1.   Cohen, S. N. Toxoplasmosis in patients receiving immunosuppression therapy. *J. A. M. A. 211*, 657 (1970).
2.   Siegel, S. E., et. al. Transmission of toxoplasma by leukocyte transfusion. *Blood 37*, 388 (1971).
3.   Stinson, E. B. Infectious complication after cardiac transplantation in man. ~~n.~~ *Int. Med. 74*, 22 (1971).
4.   Sulzer, A. J. and Hall, E. C. Indirect fluorescent antibody tests for parasitic disease. IV. Statistical study of variation in the indirect fluorescent antibody (IFA) test for toxoplasmosis. *Am. J. Epidemiol. 86*, 401 (1967).
5.   Sulzer, A. J., Wilson, M., and Hall, E. C. *Toxoplasma gondii*: Polar staining in fluorescent antibody test. *Exptl. Parasitol. 29*, 197 (1971).
6.   Vietzke, W., et al. Toxoplasmosis complicating malignancy. *Cancer 21*, 816 (1968).
7.   Walton, B. C., Benchoff, B. M., and Brooks, W. H. Comparison of the indirect fluorescent antibody test and the methylene blue dye test for detection of antibodies to *Toxoplasma gondii. Am. J. Trop. Med. 15*, 149 (1966).

IF Typing of Pneumococci. Before the introduction of sulfonamides and antibodies, it was standard practice to type pneumococci in pneumonia because treatment was based on type-specific antisera. Since then, pneumococcal typing has been neglected and is not usually done routinely. However, because of the high mortality rate (5-18%) in pneumococcal infections the problem of immunization of individuals included in the high-risk group has gained importance and with it the typing of pneumococci.

Materials

1. Pneumococci are grown on blood agar. An 18-hour culture is suspended in PBS, spread on a microscope slide, fixed in 95% alcohol for three minutes, and then rinsed in PBS.
2. Type-specific rabbit antisera and normal rabbit serum
3. Goat antiserum to rabbit γ globulins, conjugated with FITC (FITC-conjugate)
4. Phosphate-buffered saline solution (PBS), pH 7.2 (p. 205)
5. Mounting fluid (p. 110)

Method

1. Apply type-specific rabbit antisera to pneumococcal smears and incubate for 30 minutes at room temperature.
2. Wash in PBS for 20 minutes, changing PBS three times.
3. Apply FITC-conjugate and incubate for 30 minutes at room temperature.
4. Wash in PBS for 20 minutes, changing PBS three times.
5. Mount with mounting fluid and read under UV microscope.

REFERENCE

1. Wicher, K., Mlodozeniec, P., and Rose, N. R. Identification of pneumococci by immunofluorescent technique. *A. S. M. 70* Annual Meeting, Boston, April 1970.

IMMUNOPEROXIDASE PROCEDURES

Immunoperoxidase (IP) procedures are based on the use of the enzyme horseradish peroxidase as a marker to visualize antigens or antibodies both at the cellular and the subcellular levels. The histochemical reaction between peroxidase and its substrate gives an insoluble reaction product visible by light and electron microscopy. These techniques were first proposed by Nakane and Pierce (13), Avrameas and Uriel (5) and have been extensively developed by Avrameas and his group (1-4).

The increasing popularity of the IP methods is due to some disadvantages inherent in the IF procedures--that is, the lack of standardization (mainly due to the problems connected with the preparation of fluorescein-conjugated antibodies), the fading of the fluorescent reactions, and the necessity of photographs to keep records of the reactions themselves. Also, the resolution of the fluorescent microscopes is not sufficient for an accurate localization of antibodies or antigens.

In contrast, the IP methods seem easier to standardize, because the preparation of peroxidase conjugates is not complicated and in some methods can be avoided completely by the use of antibodies to peroxidase instead of chemical conjugates of peroxidase. In addition, permanent preparations can be obtained for further reference, and a conventional light microscope (instead of an expensive UV microscope) can be used, thus obtaining better definition by high-power immersion objectives. Another advantage is that IP procedures are also used in immunoelectronmicroscopy (p. 127), so that the same reagents can be utilized both for light and electron microscopy; this cannot be done with fluorescein or ferritin conjugates and is a unique characteristic of the immunoenzyme procedures.

According to the reagents employed in the reaction, IP procedures can be divided into methods based on the use of peroxidase-conjugated antibodies (peroxidase conjugate methods), methods based on the use of antibodies to peroxidase (mixed antibody method and hybrid antibody method), and methods based on the use of both peroxidase conjugates and antibodies to peroxidase (amplification antibody methods).

Peroxidase Conjugate Methods

These methods are the IP procedures most commonly employed in clinical immunology and are based on the same principles applied in IF techniques, with the difference that peroxidase and not fluorescein is conjugated to the antibodies (peroxidase conjugates). As for IF, a direct and an indirect method have been described:

(1) The direct method, in which a peroxidase-labeled antibody is applied to a preparation containing the corresponding antigen, has been utilized to detect bound immunoglobulins in kidney biopsies from patients with renal diseases (8) and in skin biopsies from patients with pemphigus, bullous pemphigoid, and SLE (10). Viral antigens have also been detected by this method (11).

(2) In the indirect method, an antigen is treated with its corresponding unlabeled antibody and the resulting antigen-antibody complex is visualized by a peroxidase conjugate directed against the immunoglobulins of the same animal species as the antibody producer whose serum is tested in the first step. Antibodies to antigen of nuclei, thyroid microsomes, skin, stomach, striated muscle, and mitochondria have been detected by this method in sera of patients with different autoimmune diseases (6, 8-10, 14, 18). The indirect method has

also been used to detect antibodies to *Treponema pallidum* in sera of syphilitic patients (14) and to localize viral antigens (12, 15, 17).

Methods Using Antibodies to Peroxidase

In these procedures antibodies to peroxidase are used instead of peroxidase conjugates. Under the conditions employed in these methods, the peroxidase in the peroxidase-antiperoxidase complexes is not inactivated. Its catalytic activity allows the histochemical localization of the enzyme and thus of the antibodies immunologically bound to it. This procedure avoids the risks of overlabeling, underlabeling, or altering the antibody during the conjugation process and the possibility of deterioration of the conjugate during storage. Other advantages are a higher sensitivity than the peroxidase conjugate methods and a reduction in difficulties of staining tissues especially for immunoelectronmicroscopy. Penetration of the reagents is made easier by the fact that their molecular size does not exceed that of an IgG molecule and can be further reduced using Fab fragments. It is obvious that in these multistep procedures adequate controls for each step must be included.

Mixed Antibody, or "Bridge," Method. The basis of this method is the use of two antibodies, the first against the test antigen and the second antibody against peroxidase produced in the same species of animal. These antibodies are joined in the reaction by a "bridge," that is, an antibody against the immunoglobulins of the animal species producing the two kinds of antibodies previously mentioned. Both a direct and an indirect method can be used, as represented schematically in Fig. 5.1.

The mixed antibody method has been employed by Avrameas (3) to detect rabbit immunoglobulins in spleen cells and by Wicker (16) for the demonstration of viral antigens. In our laboratory this procedure (both in the direct and the indirect method) is regularly employed to detect human γ globulins bound to glomeruli in human kidney biopsies and circulating antibodies to antigens of nuclei, thyroid, and skin (7). According to our experience, the mixed antibody method is particularly useful to control results obtained by the peroxidase conjugate methods and lends itself very well to parallel studies by light and electron microscopy.

Hybrid Antibody Method. This method is less lengthy than the mixed antibody procedure, because of the use of hybrid antibodies--that is, antibodies possessing a double antiprotein-antienzyme specificity prepared by special treatment of mixtures of different antibodies. Also in this procedure a direct and an indirect method are possible, as represented schematically in Fig. 5.2.

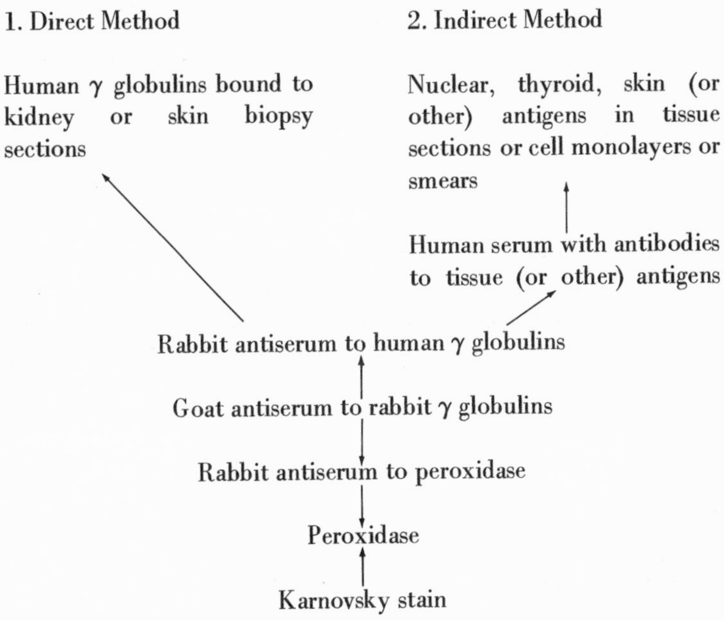

1. Direct Method   2. Indirect Method

Human γ globulins bound to   Nuclear, thyroid, skin (or
kidney   or   skin   biopsy   other) antigens in tissue
sections   sections or cell monolayers or
                                smears

                                Human serum with antibodies
                                to tissue (or other) antigens

Rabbit antiserum to human γ globulins

Goat antiserum to rabbit γ globulins

Rabbit antiserum to peroxidase

Peroxidase

Karnovsky stain

Fig. 5.1.   Schematic Representation of Mixed Antibody, or "Bridge," Method.

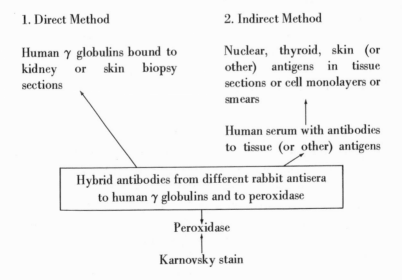

1. Direct Method   2. Indirect Method

Human γ globulins bound to   Nuclear, thyroid, skin (or
kidney   or   skin   biopsy   other) antigens in tissue
sections   sections or cell monolayers or
                                smears

                                Human serum with antibodies
                                to tissue (or other) antigens

Hybrid antibodies from different rabbit antisera
to human γ globulins and to peroxidase

Peroxidase

Karnovsky stain

Fig. 5.2.   Schematic Representation of Hybrid Antibody Method.

The hybrid antibody method has been used by Avrameas (3) for the localization of immunoglobulins in rabbit spleen cells, viral antigens in infected cells, and membrane antigens of mouse plasmocytomas.

Amplification Antibody Method

In this procedure, tissue or cells containing immunoglobulins are incubated with small amounts of peroxidase-labeled antibody to immunoglobulins, then with antiperoxidase antibody, and finally with peroxidase. According to Avrameas (3), a definite enhancement of the sensitivity of the IP reaction is thus obtained.

Peroxidase Conjugate Indirect Method for ANA

Materials

1. Mouse liver sections, cryostat-cut, 4μ, unfixed, air-dried
2. Sera from patients with SLE or other diseases and control sera (both positive and negative)
3. Peroxidase conjugate to human γ globulins (rabbit antiserum to human γ globulins, conjugated with horseradish peroxidase)
4. Karnovsky solution (p. 201)
5. Phosphate-buffered saline solution (PBS) pH 7.2 (p. 205)
6. Tris buffer 0.05M, pH 7.6
7. Graded alcohols (30, 70, 80, 95, and absolute) and xylol
8. Permanent mounting medium

Method

1. Overlay liver sections with different dilutions of sera to be tested and incubate 30 minutes at room temperature in humid chamber.
2. Rinse off sera and wash sections for 30 minutes in PBS.
3. Remove excess PBS from the slide, but make sure the tissue remains moist. Overlay sections with peroxidase conjugate appropriately diluted in PBS, and incubate 30 minutes at room temperature in humid chamber.
4. Remove and wash sections for 30 minutes in PBS.
5. Remove excess PBS from the slides, but make sure the tissue remains moist. Incubate for 6-10 minutes in Karnovsky solution.

6. Rinse in six different changes of tris buffer, then rinse in tap water once.
7. Dehydrate in graded alcohols, clear with xylol, mount with mounting medium.
8. Preparations thus obtained can be kept for a long period of time, without any appreciable change in intensity of the reaction. Positive nuclei are dark brown, while negative nuclei resemble empty vesicles against the light brown background of the cytoplasm.

Mixed Antibody Direct Method for Human γ Globulins Bound to Kidney Tissue

Materials

1. Cryostat-cut sections of human kidney biopsy, 4μ, unfixed, air-dried
2. Rabbit antiserum to human γ globulins (γ globulin fraction of rabbit antiserum)
3. Goat antiserum to rabbit γ globulins (γ globulin fraction of goat antiserum)
4. Rabbit antiserum to horseradish peroxidase (γ globulin fraction of rabbit antiserum)
5. Control sera (rabbit antiserum to γ globulins of a species other than human, goat antiserum to a species other than rabbit, rabbit antiserum to a different antigen than peroxidase, normal rabbit and goat serum)
6. Horseradish peroxidase, 0.25 mg/ml (Type VI, Sigma)
7. Karnovsky solution (p. 201)
8. Phosphate-buffered saline (PBS) solution (p. 205)
9. Tris buffer 0.05M, pH 7.6
10. Graded alcohols, xylol, and permanent mounting medium

Method

1. Overlay kidney sections with the appropriate dilution of the rabbit antiserum to human γ globulins and incubate at room temperature for 30 minutes in humid chamber. Control sections should be incubated with rabbit antiserum to γ globulins of a species unrelated to human, with normal rabbit serum and with PBS.
2. Rinse off sera and wash sections for 30 minutes in PBS.
3. Remove excess PBS from the slide, making sure the tissue remains moist.
4. Overlay sections with the appropriate dilution of goat antiserum to rabbit γ globulins and incubate at room temperature for 30 minutes in humid chamber. Different control sections should be incubated with goat anti-

serum to γ globulins of a species other than rabbit, with normal goat serum and with PBS.

5. Rinse and wash sections for 30 minutes in PBS. Then remove excess PBS from the slide, but make sure the tissue remains moist.

6. Overlay sections with the appropriate dilution of rabbit antiserum to peroxidase and incubate at room temperature for 30 minutes in humid chamber. Different control sections should be incubated with rabbit anti-serum to another antigen, with normal rabbit serum and with PBS.

7. Rinse and wash sections for 30 minutes in PBS. Then remove excess PBS from the slide, but make sure the tissue remains moist.

8. Overlay sections with the peroxidase solution and incubate at room temperature for 30 minutes in humid chamber. Different control sections should be incubated with PBS and, if desired, with another enzyme (phosphatase, etc.).

9. Rinse and wash sections for 30 minutes in PBS. Then remove excess PBS from the slides, but make sure the tissue remains moist.

10. Incubate for 6-10 minutes in Karnovsky solution, rinse in six different changes of Tris buffer, rinse once in tap water, dehydrate in graded alcohols, clear with xylol, and mount with mounting medium.

11. Preparations thus obtained can be kept for a long period of time. Deposits of γ globulin in the kidney stain dark brown.

REFERENCES

1. Avrameas, S. Coupling of enzymes to proteins with glutaraldehyde. Use of the conjugates for the detection of antigens and antibodies. *Immunochem.* 6, 43 (1969).

2. ——————. Immunoenzyme techniques: Enzymes as markers for the localization of antigens and antibodies. *Int. Rev. Cytol.* 27, 349 (1970).

3. ——————. Indirect immunoenzyme techniques for the intracellular detection of antigens. *Immunochem.* 6, 825 (1969).

4. Avrameas, S., Taudou, B., and Ternynck, T. Specificity of antibodies synthesized by immunocytes as detected by immunoenzyme techniques. *Int. Arch. Aller.* 40, 161 (1971).

5. Avrameas, S. and Uriel, J. Méthode de marquage d'antigèns et d'anticorps avec des enzymes et son application en immunodiffusion. *Compt. Rend. Ser. D*, 262, 2543 (1966).

6. Benson, M. D. and Cohen, A. S. Antinuclear antibodies in systemic lupus erythematosus. Detection with horseradish-peroxidase-conjugated antibody. *Ann. Int. Med.* 73, 943 (1970).

7.   Bigazzi, P. E., Andres, G., and Rose, N. R. Immunoperoxidase procedures. (in preparation).

8.   Davey, F. R. and Busch, G. J. Immunohistochemistry of glomerulonephritis using horseradish peroxidase and fluorescein-labeled antibody: A comparison of two techniques. *Am. J. Clin. Pathol.* *53*, 531 (1970).

9.   Dorling, J., Johnson, G. D., Webb, J. A., and Smith, M. E. Use of peroxidase-conjugated antiglobulin as an alternative to immunofluorescence for the detection of antinuclear factor in serum. *J. Clin. Path.* *24*, 501 (1971).

10. Fukuyama, K., Douglas, S. D., Tuffanelli, D. L., and Epstein, W. L. Immunohistochemical method for localization of antibodies in cutaneous disease. *Am. J. Clin. Pathol.* *54*, 410 (1970).

11. Kurstak, E., Cote, R. R., and Belloncik, S. Etude de la synthèse et de la localisation des antigènes du virus de la densonucléose (VDN) à l'aide d'anticorps conjugués à l'enzyme peroxidase ('Nouvelle méthode d'immunperoxidase). *Compt. Rend. Paris, Ser. D*, *268*, 2309 (1969).

12. Leduc, E. H., Wicker, R., Avrameas, S., and Bernhard, W. Ultrastructural localization of SV40 T antigen with enzyme-labeled antibody. *J. Gen. Virol.* *4*, 609 (1969).

13. Nakane, P. K. and Pierce, G. B. Enzyme-labeled antibodies: Preparation and application for the localization of antigens. *J. Histochem. Cytochem.* *14*, 929 (1966).

14. Petts, V. and Roitt, I. M. Peroxidase conjugates for demonstration of tissue antibodies: Evaluation of the technique. *Clin. Exptl. Immunol.* *9*, 407 (1971).

15. Siverd, N. and Sharon, N. Immunohistochemical method for detection of vaccinia virus. *Proc. Soc. Exptl. Biol. Med.* *131*, 939 (1969).

16. Wicker, R. Comparison of immunofluorescence and immunoezymatic techniques applied to the study of viral antigens. *Ann. N. Y. Acad. Sci.* *177*, 490 (1971).

17. Wicker, R. and Avrameas, S. Localization of virus antigens by enzyme-labeled antibodies. *J. Gen. Virol.* *4*, 465 (1969).

18. Wolff, K. and Schreiner, E. Ultrastructural localization of pemphigus auto-antibodies within the epidermis. *Nature* *229*, 59 (1971).

IMMUNOELECTRONMICROSCOPY

Immunoelectronmicroscopy (IEM) is a technique that allows the localization of antigens at the molecular level, using their corresponding antibodies labeled in such a way as to make them visible under the electron microscope. Antigens may be identified by using antibody conjugated with an electron-dense marker, ferritin, which can be readily recognized in the electron microscope from its characteristic appearance; or they may be localized with antibody conjugated with enzymes, like horseradish peroxidase, which can be detected histochemically. Using these, or other less frequently employed methods, the localization of surface antigens in membranes, tissue-cultured cells, or suspended cells has been accomplished, as has the identification of intracellular antigens in free cells. Studies on antigens in tissue sections have been complicated not only by the need to fix tissues for preservation of their subcellular structure while maintaining their antigenicity but also by the problem of penetration of labeled antibodies into the tissues themselves. Therefore, at present the main clinical application of IEM is the study of kidney biopsies from patients with diseases of the urinary tract. This study, which can usefully integrate the data obtained by light and fluorescence microscopy, is, of course, limited to those hospitals with an electron-microscopy unit.

Up to now, the most extensively used technique for IEM of kidney biopsies has been the immunoferritin technique. However, the immunoperoxidase technique is increasingly used, since it has the advantage of using a marker with a much lower molecular weight and therefore a much greater ease of penetration into the tissues.

Pre-embedding Staining of Kidney Biopsies with Ferritin-Conjugated Antibody

Three factors must be considered in the preparation of specimens for treatment with ferritin-conjugated antibody: the maintenance of cellular fine structure; the preservation of antigenic determinants; and the penetration of large ferritin molecules into the cells. The ideal solution to the problems would be to stain embedded thin sections directly before examining them in the electron microscope.

The usual embedding procedure, however, either greatly diminishes or eradicates the capacity of the antigen to react with antibody. The commonly used embedding polymers and the copper grids also show an electrostatic attraction that causes nonspecific binding of ferritin molecules. Consequently, the method usually employed is to prefix the specimen in reagents that do not affect the antigenic determinants but still preserve the fine structure sufficiently for electron-microscopic evaluation.

Materials

1.   Human kidney biopsies

2.   Ferritin-conjugated antibody to human γ globulins
3.   Buffered formalin (5% in PBS)
4.   Phosphate-buffered saline (PBS) solution (p. 205)
5.   Osmium tetroxide
6.   Epon 812

Method

1.   Fix kidney biopsies for 40-60 minutes at 4°C in buffered formalin and wash in cold buffer for 10 minutes.
2.   Finely mince the biopsies in the cold room using a sharp razor blade under the dissecting microscope or using a special cutting machine.
3.   Suspend the fragments in test tubes containing the ferritin conjugate for 20 minutes at room temperature with occasional agitation.
4.   After washing three times in a large volume of cold PBS, centrifuge the fragments at 3000 rpm for 10 minutes.
5.   Fix the final pellet in osmium tetroxide for 30 minutes, dehydrate in graded acetone, and embed in Epon 812.
6.   Trim the blocks and thin-section for electron-microscopy. Although not all cells are opened by the fine-cutting technique, penetration of the ferritin conjugate is sufficient to achieve satisfactory localization of γ globulins fixed to kidney tissue, while the fine structure of the kidney itself is rather well preserved.
7.   The controls routinely employed in immunoferritin studies fall into three categories: specific immunologic "blocking" of the reaction; treatment of the duplicate pieces of tissue with nonspecific ferritin conjugates; and treatment or similar, but not identical, tissue or of normal tissue with the specific ferritin conjugate.

   Blocking controls are carried out in one of two ways. In the first a piece of the kidney biopsy under study is treated with unconjugated antiserum to human γ globulin. After about 30 minutes this is washed off and the tissue is then treated with the ferritin conjugate in the same manner used for the original test. The unconjugated antibody should almost completely block the binding of the conjugated antibody. Because antigen-antibody reactions are at equilibrium, a few of the unconjugated antibodies may be replaced by conjugated antibodies. The second control test is accomplished by absorbing the specific ferritin conjugate with human γ globulin. Pieces of the kidney biopsy are tested simultaneously with the absorbed and unabsorbed ferritin conjugate. The absorbed conjugate should not be bound in the tissue.

   Treatment with ferritin-labeled antibodies not specific for human γ globulins is useful to establish the fact that the conditions of the experiment do not promote nonspecific binding of ferritin conjugates. In addition to, or in place of, the nonspecific ferritin conjugate, pure ferritin and ferritin-XC-derivative are frequently employed.

The ferritin conjugate used is also tested on normal renal tissue and also on renal tissue from patients with a renal disease other than glomerulonephritis.

REFERENCE

1.   Andres, G., Hsu, K., and Seegal, B. C. Immunologic techniques for the identification of antigens or antibodies by electron microscopy. In D. M. Weir, Ed., *Handbook of Experimental Immunology*, 2nd ed. (in preparation).

RADIOIMMUNOASSAY PROCEDURES

The availability of radioisotopes and the development of numerous procedures, both synthetic and biosynthetic, for the labeling of biochemical substrates have led to the application of tracers in a variety of analytical techniques and biological procedures. The principle of isotope dilution, which is an application of tracer materials for quantitative measurements, has been applied in the measurement of immunogenic materials. Radioimmunoassay has been developed as an immunological assay technique that takes advantage of the reactivity of an antigen for its specific antibody and the ability of the radioactive form of the antigen to compete in the reaction with an unknown concentration of the antigen. During this competitive binding, the radioactive antigen undergoes a dilution by the unknown quantity of antigen. This dilution of radioactivity can be measured and can be expressed as a function of the unknown quantity of antigen.

In a radioimmunoassay, antibodies are always present as a limiting factor. Tracer material is always present as a constant, known amount of radioactive antigen. The unknown amount of antigen and labeled antigen compete for active sites on the antibodies, and the quantity of labeled antigen-antibody complex formed is an inverse function of the unlabeled antigen concentration: the greater the amount of unlabeled antigen, the lower the radioactivity bound to the antibodies. A standard curve is prepared as each group of samples is taken for analysis. The standard curve is obtained by reacting varying known amounts of antigen with the same limiting amount of antibodies and the same constant level of radioactive antigen taken for the assay of the samples.

Radioimmunoassays require an antibody as a specific binding protein for the substance to be measured, a radioactive form of the substance reactive with the specific antibody and competitive for antibody binding sites with the nonradioactive substrate to be measured, and a method for separating the substance bound to antibody from free material. Separation of radioactivity bound to antibody from free radioactivity can be achieved by a variety of methods: (1) differential migration of the bound and free by use of chromatographic or electrophoretic techniques, (2) recovery of the free radioactivity by use of ion exchange or adsorption, or (3) recovery of the bound radioactivity by precipitation with a second antibody, inorganic salt, or organic solvent or by binding to a solid support.

Radioimmunoassays are sensitive, specific, precise, and generally rapid assays for the determination of picogram to nanogram amounts in microliter aliquots. Although originally developed for the measurement of immunogenic materials, these procedures can now be used also for many compounds generally considered nonimmunogenic as a result of the generation of antibodies by the use of conjugates of such molecules with immunogenic proteins.

Radioimmunoassay procedures are a powerful, analytical tool not only useful for the measurement of hormones but also applicable in the measurement of low-molecular-weight peptides, nucleotides, drugs, and enzymes. Radioimmunoassays have been described for a large number of substances, and in some instances complete kits are available commercially. Specific antisera and radioactive substrates can be purchased also as separate items. Among the many substances that can be determined by these procedures are: digoxin, digitoxin, adenosine $3':5'$-cyclic phosphate (cyclic AMP) and other cyclic nucleotides, angiotensin I as a measure of renin activity, angiotensin II, insulin, glucagon, human chorionic gonadotropin, prostaglandins, aldosterone, estradiol, testosterone, progesterone, gastrin, calcitonin, ACTH, triiodothyronine, morphine, luteinizing hormone, follicle-stimulating hormone, thyroid-stimulating hormone, HAA, a-fetoprotein, carcinoembryonic antigen, albumin, immunoglobulins, human fibrinopeptide A. This group represents but a partial listing, and certainly any such list will continue to grow.

Radioimmunoassay kits make available to investigators and clinicians a ready-to-use supply of antibodies, radioactive materials, and standards. The user avoids many problems of antibody production (maintenance of animals; synthesis of conjugates where required; boosting and bleeding schedules; assays for antibody titer, sensitivity, and specificity) and problems of synthesizing tracer materials (use of high levels of radioisotopes; purification techniques; assessment of binding ability). However, commercial preparation of the essential reagents at standardized levels obligates the user to follow the protocol delineated by the manufacturer of the kit. Additionally, good techniques on the part of the user in setting up a series of many tubes and in treating the usually sensitive reagents are required to attain maximal usage incorporated within a kit. Cleanliness, time, temperature, mixing of reagents and assay tubes are very important conditions.

Polystyrene tubes offer the advantage of no affinity for the antibody under the conditions of the assay and the capability for use in a centrifugation step. Reproducibility of replicates, the accuracy of the standard curve, and the results for unknowns are related to types of pipettes in use. A pipetting system is an important factor, and evaluation of a radioimmunoassay and kit components should be done with known, reliable pipettes or pipetting systems. The technique for separation of bound and free should be uniformly applied to all the tubes taken for assay. Dextran-coated charcoal offers the advantage of immediate adsorption and control of the amount of added adsorbent, but its use requires maintaining uniform suspension of the charcoal before and during pipetting. The counts per minute (cpm) that are found are dependent upon the efficiency of a counting system. A longer counting time can be taken for an instrument with a low efficiency. Increased counting times provide for better replicates and may be taken as decay of a radioactive marker occurs. However, it is important that the volume of the radioactive marker remains as described in the protocol throughout the life of the kit. This precaution also applies to the indicated volumes of other kit reagents.

Radioimmunoassay of Digoxin

Radioimmunoassay of digoxin in a small volume permits a frequent assessment of digoxin levels in patients' sera and the assay of samples from pediatric cases. The radioimmunoassay of digoxin involves the competitive binding of a radioactive digoxin derivative (3-O-succinyl digoxingenin tyrosine [^{125}I]) and circulating digoxin for antibody to digoxin. This antibody is obtained using a human-serum albumin-digoxin conjugate, is highly specific for the steroid nucleus of digoxin, and therefore shows equivalent recognition for digoxin and the digoxingenin derivative.

In the radioimmunoassay that follows, the digoxin-antibody complex forms at room temperature during an incubation time of one-half hour. The separation of bound digoxin from free digoxin is achieved by adsorption of the free digoxin, both labeled and unlabeled, on dextran-coated charcoal. After centrifugation and decantation, the bound radioactivity in the solution is determined by counting in a γ counting system. Plotting the data as percent digoxin bound against nanograms digoxin per milliliter of serum or plasma, with nanograms per milliliter as a logarithmic function, shows a linear curve in the range 1-10 ng. Since only 50 μl serum or plasma is taken per assay, linearity is demonstrated in the detection of 0.05-0.5 ng digoxin.

Materials

1. Digoxin (^{125}I) radioimmunoassay kit (Schwarz/Mann), containing digoxin standard solution, digoxin derivative (^{125}I), and digoxin antiserum
2. Serum or plasma free of radioactivity and digoxin
3. Phosphate-buffered saline (PBS) solution, pH 7.2
4. Dextran-coated charcoal (DCC) stock suspension (p. 198)
5. DCC working suspension, a 1:10 dilution of stock suspension. Maintain under magnetic stirring during subsequent use.
6. Polystyrene tubes, disposable, 12 x 75 mm (Schwarz/Mann)
7. Micropipettes, Lang-Levy, 2-, 5-, 10-, 15-, 25-, 50-μl capacities (Kimble)
8. Cornwall syringe (Bacton, Dickinson and Co.), with metal holder and tubing adapter
9. γ counting system

Method

1. Preparation of the standard curve
    A. Pipette 50 μl serum or plasma into 16 numbered tubes. Maintain the tubes at room temperature.
    B. Add 1.0 ml PBS to each tube.
    C. Add digoxin standard solution as follows:

Tube no.	Digoxin standard	Digoxin as ng/ml serum
5, 6	2 μl	0.4
7, 8	5 μl	1.0
9, 10	10 μl	2.0
11, 12	15 μl	3.0
13, 14	25 μl	5.0
15, 16	50 μl	10.0

(If desired, aliquots of the digoxin standard solution can be diluted with 30% ethanol so that 10 μl aliquots are taken in place of the 2-μl and 5-μl aliquots indicated above. For the 0.4-ng level, dilute 10 μl of standard with 40 μl 30% ethanol and for the 1.0-ng level, dilute 20 μl of standard with 20 μl of 30% ethanol. Do not prepare a dilution for these levels that will necessitate an addition to the assay in excess of 10 μl.)

D. Add 10 μl digoxin derivative (^{125}I) to tubes 1-16. Mix well.

E. Add 10 μl digoxin derivative (^{125}I) to 1.5 ml PBS in each of two polystyrene tubes numbered 17 and 18.

F. Add 10 μl digoxin antiserum to tubes 3-16.

G. Mix each tube well after each of the above additions. Shake the rack of tubes to mix all reagents thoroughly.

H. Incubate at room temperature for 30 minutes from the time of the last addition, in step F.

I. Add 0.5 ml DCC working suspension to tubes 1-16. The reagent is "squirted" into each tube to obtain a uniform suspension of charcoal in the reaction mixture, using a Cornwall syringe and metal holder with tubing adapter.

J. Keep at room temperature for five minutes from the time of the last addition, in step I.

K. Centrifuge at about 2500 rpm in the cold (about 4°C) for 20 minutes or for a time that gives adequate packing of the charcoal.

L. Decant each clear supernatant into a correspondingly numbered polystyrene tube. Maximal transfer is obtained by hitting the rims together. Discard the charcoal residues.

M. Count in the γ counter for 1-10 minutes those tubes into which the supernatants have been decanted.

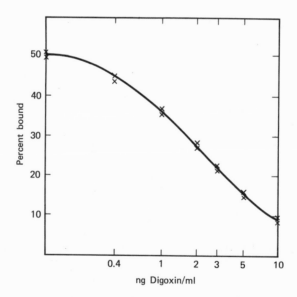

Fig. 5.3.

N. Include in the counting sequence tubes 17 and 18. The counts in these tubes should be 3000-7000 cpm; these tubes give the total count per assay.

O. Draw a standard curve on semi-logarithmic paper, percent digoxin bound against standards as nanogram per milliliter (Fig. 5.3.).

2. Clinical assays

A. Add 50 μl patient serum or plasma to each of two tubes. Keep the tubes at room temperature.

B. Add 1.0 ml PBS to each tube.

C. Add 10 μl digoxin derivative (^{125}I) to each tube.

D. Add 10 μl digoxin antiserum to each tube. Mix well.

E. Incubate at room temperature for 30 minutes.

F. Add 0.5 ml DCC working suspension to each tube, as above.

G. Keep at room temperature for five minutes from the time of the last addition, in step F.

H. Centrifuge at the same speed and for the same time used for the standards.

I. Decant each clear supernatant into a correspondingly numbered plastic tube. Discard the charcoal residues.

J. Count each tube containing the decanted solution for the same period taken for the standards.

A protocol for the assay of digoxin is shown in Table 5.1.

Table 5.1.   Protocol for Radioimmunoassay of Digoxin

Tube no.	Serum	Buffer	Standard	^{125}I	A$_b$	*	DCC
1, 2	50 μl	1.0 ml	--	10 μl	--	*	0.5 ml
3, 4	50 μl	1.0 ml	--	10 μl	10 μl	*	0.5 ml
5, 6	50 μl	1.0 ml	2 μl	10 μl	10 μl	*	0.5 ml
7, 8	50 μl	1.0 ml	5 μl	10 μl	10 μl	*	0.5 ml
9, 10	50 μl	1.0 ml	10 μl	10 μl	10 μl	*	0.5 ml
11, 12	50 μl	1.0 ml	15 μl	10 μl	10 μl	*	0.5 ml
13, 14	50 μl	1.0 ml	25 μl	10 μl	10 μl	*	0.5 ml
15, 16	50 μl	1.0 ml	50 μl	10 μl	10 μl	*	0.5 ml
17, 18	--	1.5 ml	--	10 μl	10 μl	*	--
19, 20 (patient sample)	50 μl	1.0 ml	--	10 μl	10 μl	*	0.5 ml

* 30 min. @ Room Temp.

3.   Calculations
  A.   The "blank," or "background," is the average count found in tubes 1 and 2.
  B.   Under "Preparation of the standard curve"
    (1)   The counts found in tubes 3-16 are corrected by subtracting the "blank" counts.
    (2)   The average of the counts found in tubes 17 and 18, the total count per assay, is corrected by subtracting the blank counts.
    (3)   Percent bound $= \dfrac{\text{standard count (B1)}}{\text{total count (B2)}} \times 100$
    (4)   The percent bound for tubes 3 and 4, "trace binding," indicates the binding of digoxin derivative (^{125}I) in the absence of digoxin standards.
    (5)   Plot percent bound against nanograms per milliliter of serum semi-log paper with nanograms per milliliter as the logarithmic function.
  C.   Under "Clinical assay"
    (1)   The counts found in step J. are corrected for the "blank" counts, as above.
    (2)   Percent bound $= \dfrac{\text{serum sample count (C1)}}{\text{total count (B2)}} \times 100$

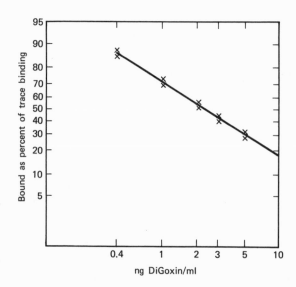

Fig. 5.4.

(3) Determine nanograms per milliliter of serum from the standard curve.

The plotting of data as percent bound versus log dosage produces a curve that is partially linearized. More complete linearization of the standard curve can be obtained with logit-log paper by plotting each percent bound as a percent of the trace binding (cpm bound in the presence of standard as a percent of the cpm bound in the absence of standard) as a logit function versus concentration as a logarithmic function. Typical semi-log and logit plots are shown in Fig. 5.3 and Fig. 5.4, respectively.

REFERENCES

1.   Berson, S. A. and Yalow, R. S. General principles of radioimmunoassay. *Clin. Chim. Acta 22*, 51 (1968).
2.   Berson, S. A. and Yalow, R. S. Radioimmunoassay: A status report. *Hosp. Prac. November*, 73-83 (1968).
3.   Herbert, V., Lau, K. Ś., Gottlieb, C. W., and Bleicher, S. J. Coated Charcoal immunoassay of insulin. *J. Clin. Endocrinol. 25*, 1385 (1965).
4.   Rodbard, D., Bridson, W., and Rayford, P. L. Rapid calculation of radioimmunoassay results. *J. Lab. Clin. Med. 74*, 770 (1969).
5.   Smith, T. W., Butler, V. P., Jr., and Haber, E. Determination of therapeutic and toxic serum digoxin concentrations by radioimmunoassay. *N. E. J. Med. 281*, 1212 (1969).
6.   Smith, T. W. and Haber, E. Digoxin intoxication: The relationship of clinical presentation to serum digoxin concentration. *J. Clin. Invest. 49*, 2377 (1970).
7.   Yalow, R. S. and Berson, S. A. Immunoassay of endogenous plasma insulin in man. *J. Clin. Invest. 39*, 1157 (1960).
8.   Yalow, R. S., Berson, S. A., et. al. Radioimmunoassay, Sessions 7 and 8. In *In Vitro Procedures with Radioisotopes in Medicine* (International Atomic Energy Agency: Vienna, 1970), p. 455.

Chapter 6

LEUKOCYTE TYPING

F. Milgrom   K. Kano

The HL-A system has been known to be a major histocompatibility system in man (1). This system can be divided into two segregant series of antigens, called the first (LA) and the second (four). Each series of antigens is governed by separate, but closely linked, loci on a pair of autosomes. Thus, each of the HL-A chromosomes carries genetic information for two antigens, one from the first and the other from the second series (10). It was also found that crossing over between these two loci occurs with a frequency of less than 1.0% (9).

Significance of HL-A serotyping in transplantation was at first documented in skin graft experiments. It was clearly shown that skin grafts exchanged between siblings with identical HL-A genotype had a long survival time, while grafts exchanged between siblings who received different HL-A chromosomes from both parents survived no longer than grafts between unrelated individuals (11, 2). In a similar way, clinical data (5-6) have shown that a vast majority of renal grafts (over 90%) originating from HL-A identical siblings had long-lasting survival (up to four years) with satisfactory kidney function. It should be stressed, however, that the validity of HL-A matching of grafts from unrelated individuals is still uncertain and requires further clarification.

Several serologic techniques are now available to detect HL-A antigens on a variety of nucleated cells (3, 4, 8). The microdroplet lymphocytotoxicity test, developed by Terasaki and his associates (7), has mostly been used for clinical tissue-typing.

MICRODROPLET LYMPHOCYTOTOXICITY TEST

Materials

1. Anti-HL-A sera (NIH Serum Bank)
2. Lymphocyte suspension, 5000 cells/μl (p. 202)

139

3.   Microtest plate (Falcon no. 3034)
4.   Mineral oil, extra heavy (Squibb)
5.   Repeating dispenser (Hamilton no. PB600-1)
6.   50 μl syringe (Hamilton 750SN, point style no. 3, 2 in. 22-gauge fixed needle)
7.   250 μl syringe (Hamilton 725SN)
8.   Rabbit complement
9.   Hank's balanced salt solution (HBSS)
10.   Eosin Y dye, 5% in water
11.   Formaldehyde, 40%, pH 7.0
12.   Microscope slide, 50 x 75 mm
13.   Inverted phase-contrast microscope with 10x objective

Method

1.   Fill each of the 60 wells of a microtest plate with a drop of mineral oil, using a Pasteur pipette. Invert the plate and shake strongly to remove most of the oil, leaving a film only. This oil film is required to prevent evaporation of reagents to be added.
2.   Fill each well with 1 μl of anti-HL-A serum using a fixed needle 50 μl microsyringe. Filled trays may be stored in a freezer. Care should be taken to wash the syringe thoroughly with HBSS between each antiserum.
3.   Using the same microsyringe equipment, add 1 μl of lymphocyte suspension to each well and incubate the plates for 30 minutes at room temperature.
4.   Add 5 μl of undiluted NRS as a source of complement (previously prepared in the cold and stored in small amounts at -70°C) using a 250-μl fixed needle microsyringe. Incubate the plates again for one hour at room temperature.
5.   Add 3 μl of 5% eosin for staining of dead cells, and two minutes later add 5 μl of formaldehyde for fixation of the cells.
6.   Cover wells with a 50 x 75 mm microscope slide.
7.   The test can be read at any time. It is most useful to use an inverted phase-contrast microscope with 10x objective. Dead cells look like dark red flat discs and appear larger than living cells. Living cells appear luminous with a darker ring surrounding them.

Semiquantitative evaluation

$\leqslant$10% dead cells: —
10-20% dead cells: ±
20-40% dead cells: +

40-70% dead cells: ++
>70% dead cells: +++

REFERENCES

1. Ceppellini, R. Facts about transplantation antigens in man. In B. D. Amos, Ed. *Progress in Immunology* (Academic: New York and London, 1971), p. 973.
2. Ceppellini, R., Bigliani, S., Curtoni, E. S., and Leigheb, G. Experimental allotransplantation in man. II. The role of A_1, A_2 and B antigens. III. Enhancement by circulating antibody. *Transplant. Proc. 1*, 385 (1969).
3. Colombani, J., Colombani, M., Benjamin, A., and Dausset, J. Leukocyte and platelet antigens defined by platelet complement fixation test. In E. S. Curtoni, P. L. Mattiuz, and R. M. Tosi, Eds., *Histocompatibility Testing* (Munksgaard: Copenhagen, 1967), p. 413.
4. Juji, T., Kano, K., and Milgrom, F. Mixed agglutination with platelets. *Int. Arch. Aller. 42*, 474 (1972).
5. Kissmeyer-Nielsen, F., Staub-Nielsen, L., Lindholm, A., Sandberg, L., Svejgaard, A., and Thorsby, E. The HL-A system in relation to human transplantation. In P. I. Terasaki, Ed., *Histocompatibility Testing* (Munksgaard: Copenhagen, 1970), p. 105.
6. Mickey, M. R., Kreisler, M., Albert, E. D., Tanaka, N., and Terasaki, P. I. Analysis of HL-A incompatibility in human renal transplants. *Tissue Antigens 1*, 57 (1971).
7. Mittal, K. K., Mickey, M. R., Singal, D. P., and Terasaki, P. I. Sero-typing for homotransplantation XVIII: Refinement of microdroplet lymphocytotoxicity test. *Transplantation 6*, 913 (1968).
8. Payne, R., Perkins, H. A., and Najarian, J. S. Compatibility for seven leukocyte antigens in renal homografts: Utilization of a micro-agglutination test with few sera. In E. S. Curtoni, P. L. Mattiuz, and R. M. Tosi, Eds., *Histocompatibility Testing* (Munksgaard: Copenhagen, 1967), p. 237.
9. Svejgaard, A., Bratlie, A., Hedin, P. J., Högman, C., Jersild, C., Kissmeyer-Nielsen, F., Lindblom, B., Lindholm, A., Löw, B., Messeter, L., Möller, E., Sandberg, L., Staub-Nielsen, L., and Thorsby, E. The recombination fraction of the HL-A system. *Tissue Antigens 1*, 81 (1971).
10. Terasaki, P. I. Joint report of the 4th International Histocompatibility Workshop. In P. I. Terasaki, Ed., *Histocompatibility Testing* (Munksgaard: Copenhagen, 1970).
11. van Rood, J. J., van Leewen, A., Schippers, A., Ceppellini, R., Mattiuz, P. L., and Curtoni, S. Leukocyte groups and their relation to homotransplantation. *Ann. N. Y. Acad. Sci. 129*, 467 (1966).

ERRATA

CHAPTER 1

Page 8 - line 15 -   8. Those plates that are to be stored........

CHAPTER 4

Page 85 - Protocol 4.3 - line 3 -
```
        group 0 non-sec.
          control
             b
```

Page 86 - line 10 -   (Ejnar Munksgaard........

CHAPTER 5

Page 132 - para. 2 - line 4 -   digoxigenin tyrosine........

Page 132 - para. 2 - line 8 -   digoxigenin derivative.

Page 133 - line 6 -   solution, pH 7.4

Page 133 - line 12 -   8. Cornwall syringe (Becton.............

Page 135 - Table 5.1 - line 9 -   17,18 – 1.5ml – 10μl – * –

Page 136 - line 14 -   (5) Plot percent bound against nanograms per milliliter
                         of serum on semi-log paper with ....

CHAPTER 7

Page 143 - para. 3 - line 3 -   standard in vivo method of ....

CELL-MEDIATED IMMUNOLOGICAL REACTIONS

S. Cohen   R. Zeschke

The population of sensitized lymphocytes which mediate delayed hypersensitivity is able to produce a variety of non-antibody effector substances when stimulated by antigen. These are collectively known as lymphokines, some of which are here listed:

Lymphokine	*Properties*
Eosinophil chemotactin	Attracts eosinophils following interaction with immune complexes
Interferon	Anti-viral activity
Lymphotoxin	Kills various nucleated target cells
Lymphocyte chemotactin	Attracts other lymphocytes
Macrophage-activation factor	Enhances macrophage motility and phagocytosis
Macrophage chemotactin	Attracts macrophages
Migration-inhibition factor (MIF)	Prevents macrophage migration in vitro
Mitogenic factor	Causes blast transformation of lymphocytes
Neutrophil chemotactin	Attracts neutrophils
Skin-reactive factor	Produces inflammatory reaction in skin
Transfer factor	Passive transfer of delayed hypersensitivity in man
Proliferation inhibition factor	Inhibits multiplication of non-lymphoid cells

For the most part, lymphokine activity has been evaluated in in vitro systems, two of which, the migration inhibition test and the lymphocyte-transformation test, have found increasing application in clinical immunology.

Even though in vitro tests are susceptible to criticism because of the removal of the cultured cells from the living environment, they nonetheless provide certain advantages over the standard in vitro method of assessing

143

cell-mediated immunity (skin-testing). Skin-testing involves the introduction of the specific antigen into the organ with the possibility of altering the immune status of the patient as well as involving many variables that are beyond appreciation and control. In transplantation studies, skin-testing may cause specific sensitization to occur; in general, quantitation of the intradermal reaction is subjective and difficult.

While the in vitro assays for delayed hypersensitivity circumvent the above drawbacks of skin-testing, it should be emphasized that in vitro assays have their own set of limitations. The assay for a specific lymphokine such as migration-inhibitory factor or blastogenic factor represents only one facet of a complex and incompletely understood process. The role of each of the dozen or more mediator substances in response to a particular pathogen and their relationship to one another is not clear at the moment. One cannot assume that each lymphokine is involved to the same extent in each instance of a delayed hypersensitivity response. Nor can one assume that these products of antigen-stimulated sensitized lymphocytes are involved only in delayed hypersensitivity. This is particularly true of mitogenic factor which promotes lymphocyte transformation; blastogenesis clearly represents an initial step of both humoral and cellular immunologic responses.

REFERENCES

1.   Bloom, B. R. and Glade, P. R. *In Vitro Methods in Cell-Mediated Immunity* (Academic: New York, 1971).
2.   Cohen, S., Cudkowicz, G., and McCluskey, R. T. *Cellular Interactions in the Immune Response* (Karger: Basel, 1971).
3.   McClusky, R. T. and Cohen, S. *Mechanisms of Cell-Mediated Immunity* (Wiley: New York, in preparation).

IN VITRO ASSAYS OF CELLULAR IMMUNITY

The first of these assays, migration inhibition, measures the production of a lymphokine (migration-inhibition factor or MIF) by its effect on a target cell population (other lymphocytes or macrophages).

The second in vitro assay, lymphocyte transformation, measures the blastogenic response of lymphocytes to specific (antigen) stimulation, nonspecific (phytohemagglutinin or PHA) stimulation, or to a lymphokine known as mitogenic factor. While the formation of large "blast" cells can be detected with a microscope, it is more convenient to determine the extent of blastogenesis by measuring the amount of a DNA precursor taken up by these cells for DNA replication. This is done by adding tritium-labeled thymidine to the medium in which the lymphocytes are cultured.

Migration Inhibition

This test measures the production of migration-inhibition factor (MIF) by its effect on a target cell population (macrophages or blood monocytes). While being conducted in vitro and representing but a single event in the cellular response, this test has gained a reputation for being an excellent and specific indicator of cellular immunity (5). The basic concept of inhibition of cell migration was developed by George and Vaughan (8) in 1962 and subsequently refined by David et al. (3-5).

This technique is based upon the observation that peritoneal exudate cells (PE cells) (approximately 75% macrophages and 20% lymphocytes) from a sensitized animal (most often a guinea pig) when packed in a capillary tube demonstrate a tendency to migrate out of that tube. This inclination to migrate can be inhibited by adding the sensitizing antigen to the medium used for incubation of the macrophage-containing tubes. The reaction of the sensitized lymphocytes in the PE cell population with antigen releases into the medium a factor, MIF, that inhibits the migration of the macrophages.

Clinically, the migration-inhibition test is beginning to find application in the assay of delayed hypersensitivity specifically with regard to autoimmunity (6, 10, 12), in the evaluation of the reconstitution of delayed hypersensitivity (8, 11), and in organ transplantation (7). It may also be used as an assay where an in vivo (serum) factor is suspected of suppressing the immune response. It is a more complex alternative to skin-testing.

Four methods have been developed for the in vitro assay of human delayed hypersensitivity based upon migration-inhibition factor. Each of these methods has its particular advantages depending upon the clinical situation.

Inhibition of Migration of Normal Guinea Pig Peritoneal Exudate Cells. This method was developed by Thor and Dray (15), who found that patients' lymphocytes cultured in the presence of an appropriate antigen released MIF into the culture medium and that the addition of this medium (after dialysis and concentration) inhibited the migration of normal guinea pig peritoneal exudate cells.

Materials

1. Patient's lymphocytes (p. 203)
2. Guinea pig peritoneal exudate cell suspension (PE cells) (p. 203)
3. Antigen
4. Tissue culture medium 199 (TC-199)
5. Penicillin G
6. Streptomycin
7. Guinea pig serum
8. Fetal calf serum
9. Siliconized 0.75-mm capillary tubes and coverslips (Note: the size of the capillary tubes is critical).
10. Mackaness-type chambers
11. Dialysis membrane (sterilized by boiling)
12. Sodium bicarbonate

Method

1. Culture patient's lymphocytes in TC-199 (3-5 x 10^6 cells/ml) in the presence of the appropriate antigen. After 24-48 hours in culture, the tubes are centrifuged and the cell-free supernatant collected. The supernatant is dialyzed under pressure against TC-199. Following concentration to one-tenth of the original volume, 10% guinea pig serum, 5% fetal calf serum, 50 units/ml penicillin, and 100 μg/ml streptomycin are added and the resultant mixture adjusted to pH 7.4 with bicarbonate. This material will be the culture medium in which the guinea pig PE cells placed in capillary tubes are cultured in Mackaness-type chambers.
2. Draw the guinea-pig-PE-cell suspension into 75-mm capillary tubes to within 1 in. of the top, and seal one end with sterile paraffin. Centrifuge the capillary tubes at approximately 100 g for five minutes and cut them 1 mm behind (cell side) the cell-fluid interface. Affix the short piece of capillary tube to the coverslip of a Mackaness-type culture chamber with sterile silicone and seal the top coverslip with sterile paraffin.
3. Fill the chamber with culture medium (from step 1), using a syringe, and seal with sterile paraffin. Incubate at 37°C for 18-24 hours.
4. Project the image of the capillary tube and migrating cells on a viewing screen and trace area of migration on paper. Determine the area of migration from the paper utilizing a planimeter. The amount of inhibition of migration is expressed by the following formula:

$$\frac{\text{Average area of migration with antigen}}{\text{Average area of migration without antigen}} \times 100 = \% \text{ migration inhibition}$$

Inhibition of Migration of Patients' Leukocytes. This method was introduced by Bendixon and Søberg (1, 14) who observed that human peripheral leukocytes from sensitized individuals are inhibited from migrating by the presence of the specific antigen in the culture medium. The technique has been modified by Rosenberg and David (13).

Materials

1. Patient's leukocytes (p. 201)
2. Horse serum
3. Hanks' balanced salt solution (HBSS)
4. Heparin (preservative free)
5. 1.4-mm capillary tubes (Note: Do not use 0.75 mm as in previous section)
6. Other materials as in previous section

Method

1. Suspend the patient's leukocytes in TC-199 with 10% horse serum. Adjust their number to a cell concentration of 7.0 x 10^7/ml and draw into capillary tubes.
2. Seal the capillary tubes, centrifuge at 2000 g for 10 minutes at 20°C, cut 1 mm below the cell-liquid interface, and place in the chambers (one capillary tube per chamber).
3. Fill the chambers with TC-199 and 10% horse serum with or without antigen, seal, and incubate for 24 hours at 37°C.
4. Results are evaluated as in previous section.

Migration Inhibition Using Human Leukocytes Combined with Guinea Pig Peritoneal Cells. Recently we (16) have found that 5-20% patient's leukocytes directly combined with guinea pig peritoneal exudate cells in capillary tubes can be used to measure MIF production. Either leukocytes or lymphocytes can be employed. This technique has the advantage of requiring only one day and as little as 4-5 ml of a patient's blood, which is of advantage in small children and lymphopenic individuals.

Materials

1. Peritoneal exudate cells (p. 203)
2. Patient's leukocytes (p. 201)
3. Other materials as in "Inhibition of Migration of Normal Guinea Pig Peritoneal Exudate Cells."

Method

1.   Combine leukocytes (pellet) with 10% volume suspension of guinea pig PE cells, so as to have 15% leukocytes by number.
2.   Proceed as in "Inhibition of . . . Exudate Cells."

Inhibition of Migration of Patients' Leukocytes in Gel. A technique for obtaining leukocyte migration in gel has been devised which is easy, quick, and utilizes techniques familiar to diagnostic laboratory personnel (2). This method requires only 5-10 ml of blood and, excluding sedimentation of the blood, takes less than one hour.

Materials

1.   Patient's leukocytes (p. 201)
2.   Disposable plastic petri dishes, 60 x 15 mm
3.   TC medium 199, 10X (Gibco)
4.   Agarose (Bausch and Lomb)
5.   Fetal calf serum
6.   Phosphate buffer
7.   Sodium bicarbonate solution 10% (Difco)
8.   Penicillin G and streptomycin
9.   Hemocytometer and diluting pipettes

Method

1.   Combine agarose, fetal calf serum, and TC-199 at 47°C to obtain 0.75% agarose and 10% fetal calf serum in 1X TC-199. To this add 50 units/ml penicillin and 50 μg/ml streptomycin. After incubation in 2% CO_2 and 98% air saturated with H_2O (in a CO_2 incubator), add sodium bicarbonate to adjust the pH to 7.2-7.4.
2.   Pour five ml of the agar-serum-TC-199 mixture into each plate and after solidification punch 8 to 12 holes, 2.3 mm, into the gel.
3.   Draw 10-20 ml blood in 1000 units of preservative free heparin.
4.   Allow red blood cells to sediment in the syringe (point up, inclined at an angle of 45°) at 37°C for one half hour to one hour.
5.   Place a new needle on the syringe, bend it to a 90° angle and remove buffy coat into a sterile test tube.
6.   Centrifuge at 300 g for 5 minutes, and wash cell pellet in HBSS two times.
7.   Add TC medium 199 with 10% serum to give about 2 x 10^8 cells/ml (the volume will be less than 0.5 ml).

8. Divide the leukocyte suspension into two equal parts, and add antigen in phosphate buffer to one part and an equal volume of phosphate buffer to the other. Incubate the cells for 30-60 minutes at 37°C.

9. Add seven ml of the leukocyte suspension (7 x 10^6 leukocytes) to each well.

10. Incubate the plates in 2% CO_2 and 98% air saturated with H_2O at 37°C for 24 hours. It is critical that the plates be absolutely level during incubation.

11. Determine the results by measuring the area of migration (p. 146).

REFERENCES

1. Bendixen, G. and Søborg, M. Comments on the leukocyte migration as an in vitro method for demonstrating cellular hypersensitivity in man. *J. Immunol. 104*, 1551 (1970).

2. Clausen, I. E. Tuberculin-induced migration inhibition of human peripheral leukocytes in agarose medium. *Acta Allerg. 26*, 56 (1971).

3. David, J. R., Lawrence, H. S., and Thomas, L. Delayed hypersensitivity in vitro. I. The specificity of inhibition of cell migration by antigens. *J. Immunol. 93*, 264 (1964).

4. —————————. Delayed hypersensitivity in vitro. II. Effect of sensitive cells on normal cells in the presence of antigen. *J. Immunol. 93*, 279 (1964).

5. —————————. Delayed hypersensitivity in vitro. III. The specificity of hapten protein conjugates in the inhibition of cell migration. *J. Immunol. 93*, 279 (1964).

6. David, J. H. and Paterson, P. Y. In vitro demonstration of cellular sensitivity in allergic encephalomyelitis. *J. Exptl. Med. 122*, 1161 (1955).

7. Eddleston, A. L. W. F., Williams, R., and Calne, R. Y. Cellular immune response during the rejection of liver transplant in man. *Nature 222*, 674 (1969).

8. George, M. and Vaughan, J. H. In vitro cell migration as a model for delayed hypersensitivity. *Proc. Soc. Exptl. Biol. Med. 111*, 514 (1962).

9. Levin, A. S., Spitler, L. E., Stites, D. P., and Fudenberg, H. H. Wiskott-Aldrich syndrome, a genetically determined cellular immunologic deficiency: Clinical and laboratory response to therapy with transfer factor. *Proc. Nat. Acad. Sci. 67*, 821 (1970).

10. Rauch, H., Ferraresi, R. W., Raffel, S., and Einstein, E. R. Inhibition of in vitro cell migration in experimental allergic encephalomyelitis. *J. Immunol. 102*, 1431 (1969).

11. Rocklin, R. E., Chilgren, R. A., Hong, R., and David, J. R. Transfer of

cellular hypersensitivity in chronic mucocutaneous candidiasis monitored in vivo and in vitro. *Cell. Immunol. 1*, 290 (1970).

12. Rocklin, R. E., Sheremata, W. A., Feldman, R. G., Kies, M. W., and David, J. R. Cellular response in Guillain-Barré and multiple sclerosis. *N. E. J. Med. Med. 284*, 803 (1971).

13. Rosenberg, S. A. and David, J. R. Inhibition of leukocyte migration: An evaluation of the in vitro assay of delayed hypersensitivity in man to soluble antigen. *J. Immunol. 105*, 1447 (1970).

14. Søborg, M. and Bendixen, G. Human lymphocyte migration as a parameter of hypersensitivity. *G. Acta Medica Scand. 181*, 247 (1967).

15. Thor, D. E. and Dray, S. A correlate of human delayed hypersensitivity: Specific inhibition of capillary tube migration of sensitized human lymph node cells by tuberculin and histoplasmin. *J. Immunol. 101*, 51 (1968).

16. Zeschke, R. H. and Provost, T. T. An assay technique for MIF in humans using guinea pig macrophages and human lymphocytes (submitted for publication).

Lymphocyte Transformation

Lymphocyte transformation is not as specific an indicator of delayed hypersensitivity as is migration inhibition. It has been shown that rabbits sensitized with chicken red blood cells in a fashion that will result in circulating antibody production and not in delayed hypersensitivity will exhibit lymphocyte transformation (9). There is additional evidence that lymphocytes that have undergone transformation in response to a specific antigen synthesize antibody to that antigen (2).

In addition to reflecting the ability to produce a humoral response, there is evidence that lymphocyte transformation may be an excellent method of determining the sensitivity of atopic patients (3-4). It would appear that the small lymphocytes that initially transform in the presence of a specific antigen are memory cells that may play a role in various immunological responses (1, 13, 17).

In certain conditions characterized by impaired delayed hypersensitivity but normal antibody production, lymphocyte transformation in the presence of a nonspecific mitogen (PHA, pokeweed, etc.) may be abnormally low. Such conditions are Hodgkin's disease (6), sarcoidosis (7), Sjögren's syndrome (11), and certain congenital disorders such as Swiss agammaglobulinemia (8), ataxia telangiectasia (10, 14), DiGeorge's syndrome (12), and the Wiskott-Aldrich syndrome (15). The role played by lymphocytes in congenital disorders has been reviewed by Gotoff (5).

In addition, lymphocyte transformation may be used to measure a patient's response to specific antigens (e.g., PPD, *Monilia*), to tissue and organ antigens, or in conjunction with a sensitizing agent such as DNCB or DNFB.

Finally, relating back to nonspecific stimulation as a means of assessing the general well-being and responsiveness of lymphocytes, lymphocyte transformation may be used to measure the effect of antilymphocytic agents (e.g., ALS).

Materials

1. Phytohemagglutinin-P (PHA-P) (Difco)
2. Tritiated thymidine (TdR^{3}H), specific activity 2000 mCi/mM (Amersham-Searle, Des Plaines, Ill.)
3. Culture medium TC-199 (Grand Island Biologicals, Buffalo)
4. Preservative-free heparin (Abbott Labs, Chicago)
5. Culture tubes, 17 x 100 mm (Falcon)
6. 2,5-diphenyloxazole (PPO, Amersham-Searle)
7. 1,4-bis-2-(5-phenyloxazolyl)-benzene (POPOP, Amersham-Searle)
8. NCS solubilizer (Amersham-Searle)
9. Trichloracetic acid (TCA, Amersham-Searle)
10. Sodium hydroxide, 0.1N

Method

1. Setting up cultures
    A. Draw 20 cc blood in 2000 units of preservative-free heparin.
    B. Sediment for approximately one-half hour at 37°C.
    C. Remove plasma containing leukocytes and centrifuge at 250 g for five minutes.
    D. Remove and discard plasma.
    E. Add 10 ml media (TC-199), resuspend cells, and recentrifuge.
    F. Remove media, resuspend cells in 10 ml fresh media, and count in hemocytometer.
    G. Dilute suspended cells to 1 x 10^6/ml in media and culture in tubes containing 2 ml.
    H. Cultures are set up in triplicate on day 1. For PHA-stimulated cultures (0.0002 PHA-P/ml), Tdr^{3}H (1 μCi/ml) is added on day 2 and the cultures terminated on day 3.
    I. Antigen-stimulated cultures (e.g., *Candida*) are pulsed with TdR^{3}H on day 4 and the cultures terminated on day 5.
2. Preparation of cultures for scintillation counting
    A. Centrifuge cultures at 500 g for 10 minutes.
    B. Aspirate supernatant and add 2.5 ml double-distilled water to each tube; freeze at −20°C overnight.

     C.   Transfer to glass tubes and add 2.5 ml 10% cold TCA (final concentration 5 ml of 5% TCA) and mix.

     D.   After 10 minutes, centrifuge at 4°C at 500 g for 10 minutes and discard supernatant.

     E.   Add 0.5 ml of 0.1N NaOH and mix.

     F.   Add 4.5 ml of 6.7% TCA; mix and let stand for 10 minutes.

     G.   Centrifuge at 500 g at 4°C for 10 minutes and discard supernatant.

     H.   Repeat E-F and place in refrigerator overnight to precipitate.

     I.   Centrifuge for 10 minutes at 500 g at 4°C and discard supernatant.

     J.   Add 0.5 ml NCS solubilizer and mix.

     K.   Add 5 ml fluor to tube and transfer contents to counting vial (fluor: 6 g PPO and 0.05 g POPOP/l toluene).

3.   Procedure for morphological determination of blastogenesis

     A.   Same procedure as 1. above except no TdR^3H added.

     B.   At termination of cultures the tubes are centrifuged at 300 g for 10 minutes, the supernatant is discarded, and the pellet is spread on a slide and fixed in absolute ETOH for 10 minutes.

     C.   The slides are stained with acetic orcein and 500-1000 cells counted and classified as transformed or normal.

Simplified Lymphocyte Transformation Test. Ferket, et al. have examined the possibility of using small quantities of whole blood in a lymphocyte transformation test. This test requires only 2 or 3 ml of blood which may be obtained from a finger puncture. The use of whole blood from a finger puncture simplifies the initial steps of the lymphocyte transformation test, enhancing its clinical applicability. The following is a modification of the test as originally described.

Materials

1.   Microblood collecting tubes (Microcaraway, volume 0.370 ml)
2.   Hanks' balanced salt solution (HBSS)
3.   TC-199 (Gibco)
4.   Penicillin and streptomycin
5.   Conical glass centrifuge tubes
6.   Scintillation counter
7.   Trichloracetic acid
8.   NaOH
9.   NCS solubilizer (Amersham-Searle)
10. PPO and POPOP fluors (Amersham-Searle)

Method

1. Following finger puncture, six or more aliquots of blood are obtained in a sterile, heparized blood collecting tube (volume 0.370 ml). Each aliquot is emptied into a sterile, conical centrifuge tube containing 3 ml of TC-199 containing 15 units heparin/ml.
2. Add antigen or a non-specific mitogen such as PHA dissolved in 0.5 ml HBSS to duplicate tubes and HBSS to the controls. Penicillin (50 units/ml) and streptomycin (50 mg/ml) may be added, providing there is no indication of drug allergy.
3. The tubes may be cultured with the tops loose in 2% CO_2 and 98% air saturated with water. The tubes may also be sealed and cultured at 37°C.
4. [See H and I of previous section: Preparation of cultures for scintillation counting.]All procedures are carried out in the tubes in which the cells were cultured.
   A. Centrifuge cultures at 500 g for 10 minutes.
   B. Wash 2X in ice cold HBSS.
   C. Add 5 ml 1% cold acetic acid. Centrifuge for one hour at 4°C.
   D. Follow steps of section 2, Preparation of cultures for scintillation counting (p. 152), beginning at E.

REFERENCES

1. Dutton, R. W. In vitro studies of immunological response of lymphoid cells. *Advanc. Immunol. 6*, 253 (1967).
2. Elves, M. W., Roath, S., Taylor, G., and Israëls, M. C. G. The in vitro production of antibody lymphocytes. *Lancet 1*, 1292 (1963).
3. Ferket, H., Leclercq, J., and Geubelle, F. A simplified procedure for the use of the "blast-like transformation" of lymphocytes in culture as a routine clinical test. Results in a group of allergic children. *Acta Allerg. 26*, 191 (1971).
4. Girard, J. P., Rose, N. R., Kunz, M. L., Kobayashi, S., and Arbesman, C. E. In vitro lymphocyte transformation in atopic patients: Induced by antigens. *J. Aller. 39*, 65 (1967).
5. Gotoff, S. P. Lymphocytes in congenital immunological deficiency diseases. *Clin. Exptl. Immunol. 3*, 843 (1968).
6. Hersh, E. M. and Oppenheim, J. J. Impaired in vitro lymphocyte transformation in Hodgkin's disease. *N. E. J. Med. 273*, 1006 (1965).
7. Hirschhorn, K., Schreibmann, R. P., Back, F. H., and Siltzback, L. E. In vitro studies of lymphocytes from patients with sarcoidosis and lympho-

proliferative diseases. *Lancet 2*, 842 (1964).
8. Hitzig, W. H., Kay, H. E. M., and Collier, H. Familial lymphopenia with agammaglobulinemia. *Lancet 2*, 151 (1965).
9. Jevitz, M. A. and Ekstedt, R. D. Correlation of lymphocyte transformation with the in vivo immune responsiveness of rabbits. *J. Immunol. 106*, 494 (1971).
10. Leikin, S. L., Bazelon, M., and Park, K. I. In vitro lymphocyte transformation in ataxia telangiectasia. *J. Pediat. 68*, 477 (1966).
11. Leventhal, B. G., Waldorf, D. S., and Talal, N. Impaired lymphocyte transformation and delayed hypersensitivity in Sjögren's syndrome. *J. Clin. Invest. 46*, 1338 (1967).
12. Lischner, H. W., Punnett, H. H., and DiGeorge, A. M. Lymphocytes in congenital absence of thymus. *Nature 214*, 580 (1967).
13. Nowell, P. C. Unstable chromosome changes in tuberculin-stimulated cultures from irradiated patients. Evidence for immunologically committed, long-lived lymphocytes in human blood. *Blood 26*, 798 (1965).
14. Oppenheim, J. J., Barlow, M., Waldmann, T. A., and Block, J. B. Impaired in vitro lymphocyte transformation in patients with ataxia telangiectasia. *Brit. Med. J. 2*, 336 (1966).
15. Oppenheim, J. J., Balaese, R. M., and Waldmann, T. A. The transformation of normal and Wiskott-Aldrich lymphocytes by non-specific, leukocyte, bacterial, protein, and carbohydrate stimulants. *Clin. Res. 17*, 357 (1969).
16. Richter, M. and Naspitz, C. K. The in vitro blastogenic response of lymphocytes of ragweed sensitive individuals. *J. Aller. 41*, 140 (1968).
17. Vischer, T. L. and Stastny, P. Time of appearance and distribution of cells capable of secondary immune response following primary immunization. *Immunol. 12*, 675 (1967).

IN VIVO ASSAYS FOR LYMPHOKINES:
THE MACROPHAGE-DISAPPEARANCE REACTION

Except for the skin test, there is no in vivo assay for lymphokines in the human. However, the macrophage disappearance reaction (MDR) can be used in the experimental animal as an in vivo test for lymphokines.

Nelson and Boyden (3-4) were the first to observe that the injection of tuberculin into BCG-vaccinated guinea pigs caused the virtual disappearance of macrophages from the peritoneal exudate induced by the intraperitoneal administration of glycogen. This observation has been confirmed using other antigens and other animal species (1-2). The MDR is observed whether the antigen is injected intravenously, subcutaneously, or intraperitoneally, but the intraperitoneal route requires smaller amounts of antigen and is effective in a shorter time. The reaction is sensitive (positive results can be obtained with as little as 0.1 μg of PPD) and specific and parallels positive skin reactions. Sonozaki and Cohen (5-6) have demonstrated that the MDR may be passively transferred by lymphocytes or by a soluble lymphocyte-derived factor.

Materials

1. Egg albumin (Pentex)
2. Shellfish glycogen (Sigma)
3. Complete Freund's adjuvant (Difco)
4. TC-199 (Gibco)
5. Phosphate-buffered saline (PBS), pH 7.4
6. Hartley-strain guinea pigs, 400-500 g

Method

1. In immunized animals
    A. Immunize guinea pigs with egg albumin emulsified in complete Freund's adjuvant (20 μg per footpad). Skin-test with 20 μg egg albumin in PBS one week prior to use, both to check reactivity and to boost.
    B. Induce peritoneal exudates by the intraperitoneal injection of 10 ml of a sterile solution of Shellfish glycogen (0.04 mg/ml). Allow four days before MDR is to be performed.
    C. Inject intraperitoneally each experimental animal with 20 μg egg albumin in 1 ml of PBS and each control animal with 1 ml PBS.
    D. Five hours later, collect peritoneal exudates using a total volume of 40 ml PBS containing 10 units heparin/ml. Total cell counts are then performed in the same manner as routine blood counts, using a hemocytometer. Giemsa-stained smears of the exudate are examined to obtain a differential count of lymphocytes, macrophages, and granulocytes. The total number of macrophages in the exudates from each guinea pig is obtained from the total cell count and the percent macrophages present. The percent macrophage loss is then calculated from the difference between the average count for that cell type in the exudates of the control animals and in the exudates of the animals that received antigen.
2. In unimmunized animals
    A. Sensitized cells are obtained from teased lymph nodes or peritoneal exudates from donors immunized as described above. Results are most

clear-cut when purified populations of lymphocytes are used for transfer, to avoid introducing additional macrophages into the peritoneal exudates of the recipient animals. Purification of the donor cells may be accomplished by a variety of techniques; we prefer passage through glass-bead columns, according to the method of Terasaki. This leads to populations of cells consisting of over 99% lymphocytes, and of these, approximately 95-96% are small lymphocytes.

B.   Unimmunized guinea pigs are treated with glycogen as described in 1B.

C.   Four days later, animals receive an intraperitoneal injection of from 1 to 2 x 10^6 sensitized lymphocytes and 20-40 μg of antigen in Medium 199. Controls receive an equal number of cells but no antigen. Exudates are collected and examined as described above.

By either technique, one may demonstrate up to a 95% loss in peritoneal macrophages in actively or passively sensitized guinea pigs. The reaction is maximal at 4-6 hours, but positive results may be obtained anywhere from 2-24 hours.

REFERENCES

1.   Bültmann, B., Bigazzi, P. E., Heymer, B., and Haferkamp, O. Peritoneal macrophage disappearance in the rat. *Z. Immun.-Forsch. 142*, 267 (1971).
2.   Nelson, D. S. *Macrophages and Immunity* (Wiley: New York, 1969).
3.   Nelson, D. S. and Boyden, S. V. The effect of tuberculin on the peritoneal macrophages of normal and BCG vaccinated guinea pigs and mice. *Med. Res. 1*, 20 (1961).
4.   —————————. The loss of macrophages from peritoneal exudates following the injection of antigens into guinea pigs with delayed-type hypersensitivity. *Immunol. 6*, 264 (1963).
5.   Sonozaki, H. and Cohen, S. The macrophage disappearance reaction: Mediation by a soluble lymphocyte-derived factor. *Cell. Immunol. 2*, 341 (1971).
6.   —————————. The effect of sensitized lymphocytes on peritoneal exudate macrophages in the guinea pig. *J. Immunol. 106*, 1404 (1971).

Chapter 8

MISCELLANEA

C. J. van Oss   B. Rabin
H. Fuji   J. Kite
K. Wicher

PHAGOCYTOSIS

When bacteria succeed in penetrating the external membranes of the body, cellular defense mechanisms are immediately brought into play. Phagocytic blood cells, polymorphonuclear neutrophils, migrate by amoeboid movement into the infected tissue, where they ingest and destroy the bacteria if conditions are favorable.

Phagocytosis is a complex phenomenon, involving three variables: the particle ingested, the phagocytic cell, and the medium in which the process takes place. The nature and condition of each profoundly affect the efficiency of the overall process. Encapsulated bacteria are at first poorly phagocytized by neutrophils, while noncapsulated (avirulent) bacteria and inert particles such as polystyrene beads are ingested relatively quickly. This is one of the major reasons for the greater pathogenicity of encapsulated organisms. The capsulated structures, consisting of hydrophilic gels, present a surface that is not easily seized by the somewhat less hydrophilic polymorphonuclear leukocytes (5).

A number of serum factors are known to play an active role in phagocytosis. Both heat-stable and heat-labile opsonins are necessary. The former are, generally speaking, specific antibodies to surface antigens of the microorganisms, while the heat-labile opsonins are complement factors (C 1, 4, 2 and 3). Complement need not be added to the system, for there generally seems to be enough C bound to the neutrophil membrane to facilitate phagocytosis. The presence of calcium and magnesium is necessary for phagocytosis (7). The phagocytosis of encapsulated bacteria is retarded by the time-lapse involved in the formation of specific anticapsule antibodies that destroy the phagocytic inhibiting properties. (6). Inert particles and noncapsulated bacteria, on the other hand, are capable of being opsonized even by aspecific immunoglobulins and need not wait for the

157

formation of specific factors. This explains their rapid phagocytosis (5, 7).

A large number of normal peripheral neutrophil leukocytes rapidly reduce nitroblue tetrazolium (NBT) during in vitro phagocytosis of latex particles, while a smaller proportion of neutrophils is capable of reducing this dye without challenge. Neutrophils from patients with fatal granulomatous disease of childhood do not reduce NBT during in vitro phagocytosis of latex particles and have a diminished ability to destroy bacteria. On the other hand, the percentage and absolute number of neutrophils that reduce NBT are strikingly increased during bacterial infections in those subjects whose phagocytosis system is normal. For these reasons both the NBT test and the NBT-phagocytosis test are increasingly utilized in the diagnosis of bacterial infections and of granulomatous disease of childhood (1-4).

In Vitro Phagocytosis Test (5-7)

Materials

1. Suspensions of *Staphylococcus epidermidis* and *Staphylococcus epidermidis* coated with pooled human IgG (7)
2. Patient's blood
3. Sterile Hank's balanced salt solution (HBSS) containing 1% human albumin
4. Molten paraffin wax
5. Mackaness culture chambers
6. Cleaned round glass coverslips
7. Sterile blood lancets and butterfly swabs
8. Sterile 2.50-ml syringe fitted with a 26G ½ in. needle

Method

1. Cleanse tip of patient's finger thoroughly with a gauze sponge soaked with 70% alcohol. Puncture skin of finger forcefully with sterile blood lancet. Wipe off the first drop of blood with clean gauze. Apply pressure to finger from base toward nail forcing blood through the puncture wound. Deposit three or four drops of fresh fingerprick blood on the surface of a clean coverslip.
2. Place the coverslips on a moist chamber at 37°C and incubate for 25 minutes.
3. Transfer the coverslips from the incubator to a petri dish containing saline (37°C); gently agitate until the clot floats clear of the glass surface. Continue this process until most of the residual red blood cells and fibrin

are removed.

4. Each coverslip is removed with as much saline as possible and inverted into its place on the Mackaness chamber prepared in advance. Dry the outer surface with a paper towel and quickly seal it into position with molten paraffin.

5. Fill the resulting chamber with HBSS (37°C), leaving no air bubbles. Invert the chamber and incubate at 37°C for 15 minutes.

6. Drain the chambers and refill with a standardized suspension of bacteria or particles and incubate as in step 5.

7. Disassemble the chamber on a towel saturated with disinfectant. Gently wash the coverslips containing the monolayer in 37°C HBSS and allow to air-dry.

Note: *Do not blot dry! The cell side must face up.*

8. Fix the coverslips to microscopic slides with permanent mounting fluid, with the monolayer on the exposed surface, and Gram stain.

Note: *Do not heat-fix the film.*

9. Examine under oil immersion and count a total of 30-50 neutrophils; record the number of phagocytized bacteria or particles in each. The percentage of neutrophils that have engulfed bacteria or particles is the "phagocytic index," and the average number of particles per positive cell is expressed as the "mean avidity index." The product of these two indices gives the mean of number of particles ingested per phagocytic cell.

Nitroblue Tetrazolium Phagocytosis Test

Materials

The same materials used above will be used here, with the addition of the following:

1. Nitroblue tetrazolium stain
2. Latex particles (0.8 μ diameter, 2 x 10^8 particles/ml), coated with 1% pooled human γ globulin
3. Methyl green stain

Method

1. The same procedure described above is followed (using patient's as well as

normal neutrophils), up to step 5.

2.   Draw 0.14 ml HBSS from the chamber and add 0.14 ml of the nitroblue tetrazolium stain in phosphate buffer, pH 7.0.

3.   Mix by inverting chamber a few times and allow to stand at room temperature for one and a half to two minutes.

4.   Add latex particles, incubate at 37°C for 15 minutes.

5.   Take apart chamber and counterstain the coverslip containing the monolayer of neutrophils with methyl green stain for three minutes.

6.   Mount coverslip on a microscope and observe. Only cells (neutrophils or mononuclear cells) showing at least five phagocytized latex particles are counted. These are counted positive if a deep blue, somewhat granular precipitate appears to be distributed in the cytoplasm separate from engulfed particles. Often large masses of precipitate dye are present, but even slight indication of such on focusing up and down is interpreted as a positive reaction.

REFERENCES

1.   Balhner, R. L., and Nattran, D. G. Quantitative nitroblue tetrazolium test in chronic granulomatous disease. *N. E. J. Med.* 278, 971 (1968).

2.   Matula, G. and Paterson, P. Y. Spontaneous in vitro reduction of nitroblue tetrazolium by neutrophils of adult patients with bacterial infections. *N. E. J. Med.* 285, 311 (1971).

3.   Park, B. H. The use and limitations of the nitroblue tetrazolium test as a diagnostic aid. *J. Ped.* 78, 376 (1971).

4.   Park, B. H., Fikrig, S. M., and Smithwick, E. M. Infection and nitroblue tetrazolium reduction by neutrophils. *Lancet 2*, 532 (1968).

5.   van Oss, C. J. and Gillman, C. F. Phagocytosis as a surface phenomenon. I. Contact angles and phagocytosis of non-opsonized bacteria. *J. Reticuloendoth. Soc. 12*, 283 (1972).

6.   —————————. Phagocytosis as a surface phenomenon. II. Contact angles and phagocytosis of encapsulated bacteria before and after opsonization by specific antiserum and complement. *J. Reticuloendoth. Soc. 12*, 497 (1972).

7.   van Oss, C. J. and Stinson, M. W. Immunoglobulins as aspecific opsonins. I. The influence of polyclonal and monoclonal immunoglobulins on the in vitro phagocytosis of latex particles and staphylococci by human neutrophils. *J. Reticuloendoth. Soc. 8*, 397 (1970).

HEMOLYTIC PLAQUE TECHNIQUE

The hemolytic plaque technique is a method devised by Jerne and his colleagues for detecting and enumerating individual antibody-forming cells in vitro (3-5). In this assay, lymphoid cells from an animal immunized with sheep erythrocytes are incorporated in an agar layer, together with a high concentration of the sheep erythrocytes. Each lymphoid cell that releases hemolytic antibody will have sensitized red blood cells in its vicinity. Addition of complement will cause the lysis of the sensitized red blood cells localized around the antibody-forming cell. These local areas of hemolysis are termed plaques.

This technique permits the recognition and quantitation of small numbers of individual antibody-forming cells present among millions of cells that do not produce this antibody. Various modifications have been introduced that extend the technique to antigens other than red blood cells (1, 2, 6-8). The technique described below is designed to measure high efficiency IgM hemolytic antibodies. The IgG antibodies, which are of lower hemolytic efficiency, require addition to the plate of an antiglobulin reagent, constituting the so-called indirect hemolytic plaque technique.

Materials

1. Mice, normal and immunized with sheep red blood cells
2. Agar
3. Sheep red blood cells (SRBC)
4. Phosphate-buffered saline (PBS), pH 7.2
5. Sterile petri dishes, 60 x 15 mm and 100 x 15 mm
6. 2X and 1X Eagle's minimum essential medium (MEM) in Hank's balanced salt solution (HBSS)
7. Benzidine solution for staining agar plates (0.2 gm benzidine dihydrochloride, 90 ml distilled water, 10 ml glacial acetone acid, and 0.5 ml 30% hydrogen peroxide). The solution is stored at 4-6°C.
8. Nuclear stain (0.1% crystal violet in 0.1M citric acid)
9. DEAE dextran solution (10 mg/ml in 1X Eagle's medium). DEAE dextran is necessary only to overcome the anticomplementary effect of certain preparations of agar. It should not be required with good quality agar.
10. Humidified 37°C incubator that contains an atmosphere consisting of 5% carbon dioxide in air
11. Wassermann tubes

Method

1.   Preparation of spleen-cell suspensions
    A.   Remove spleen from a normal mouse and a mouse immunized four days previously with 4×10^8 SRBC.
    B.   Weigh each spleen to nearest milligram and place it in a 60 x 15 mm petri dish containing 2.5 ml cold MEM.
    C.   Disrupt each spleen by scraping against a 50-mesh stainless-steel grid.
    D.   Filter each suspension through a 200-mesh stainless-steel grid and collect it in a graduated centrifuge tube. Keep the cell suspension on ice.
    E.   Add sufficient MEM to the suspensions so that the final volumes for the normal and the immune spleen cell suspension are 2.5 and 10 ml, respectively.
    F.   Place 0.1 ml of the suspension of normal spleen cells in 3.9 ml of the nuclear stain and 0.1 ml of the suspension of immune spleen cells in 0.9 ml of the stain.
    G.   Keep these two tubes at room temperature, and after the plates are set up, determine the number of nucleated cells per milliliter in a hemocytometer.
2.   Preparation of plates with agar-base layer
    A.   Prepare 2.8% agar by adding 2.8 gm agar to 100 ml of distilled water.
    B.   Autoclave the mixture at 121°C for 20 minutes to dissolve the agar and cool the agar solution to 45°C.
    C.   Warm 100 ml of 2X Eagle's MEM to 45°C.
    D.   Add the warm medium to the agar solution and mix well. This gives a solution of 1.4% agar in 1X Eagle's MEM.
    E.   Dispense 10 ml of the above solution into twenty 100 x 15 mm petri dishes. Allow the agar to solidify and remove the lid.
    F.   Place in a 37°C incubator for one hour with the top side down.
    G.   Replace lid and store at 4°C until needed.
    H.   Before use, bring plates to room temperature.
3.   Plating of spleen cells
    A.   Prepare 1.4% agar by adding 0.7 gm agar to 50 ml of distilled water and boil to dissolve. Cool to 45°C.
    B.   Mix agar solution with an equal volume of 2X Eagle's MEM prewarmed to 45°C.
    C.   For each spleen-cell suspension to be assayed, place two Wassermann test tubes in the 45°C waterbath.
    D.   Add 0.1 ml DEAE solution to each tube.
    E.   Place 2 ml of the agar solution prepared in step B into each Wasser-

mann tube.

F. To each Wassermann tube, add 0.1 ml of 20% SRBC.

G. Add to proper tubes 0.8 ml of normal-spleen-cell suspension or 0.05 ml of immune-spleen-cell suspension.

H. Mix the contents by rotating the tube between the palms of the hands and pour the contents of each Wassermann tube into a previously prepared agar plate. Spread the agar evenly by gently rotating the plate.

I. Allow the agar to solidify and incubate for one hour at 37°C in the carbon dioxide incubator.

J. After incubation, add to each plate 2 ml of fresh guinea pig serum diluted 1:10 in PBS.

K. Place in the carbon dioxide incubator for an additional 30 minutes.

L. Remove the plates and keep at room temperature for one to two hours.

M. Stain plates with benzidine immediately or store overnight at 4°C and stain the next morning.

4. Staining the plates

A. Add 2 ml of the benzidine stain to each plate.

B. When agar assumes a blue color, wash off stain with saline.

C. Plates may be kept at 4°C for several days after staining.

5. Counting the plaques: Plaques that appear as clear areas in the agar are conveniently counted by inspecting the plate under a dissecting microscope.

REFERENCES

1. Fuji, H., Zaleski, M., and Milgrom, F. Allogenic nucleated cells as immunogen and target for plaque-forming cells in mice. *Transplant. Proc. 3*, 852 (1971).

2. Golub, E. S., Mishell, R. I., Weigle, W. O., and Dutton, R. W. A modification of the hemolytic plaque assay for use with protein antigens. *J. Immunol. 100*, 133 (1968).

3. Jerne, N. K. and Nordin, A. A. Plaque formation in agar by single antibody producing cells. *Science 140*, 405 (1963).

4. Jerne, N. K., Nordin, A. A., and Henry, C. The agar-plaque technique for recognizing antibody producing cells. In B. Amos and H. Koprowski, Eds., *Cell Bound Antibodies* (Wistar Institute: Philadelphia, 1963).

5. Jerne, N. K., Nordin, A. A., Henry, C., Fuji, H., and Koros, A. The agar-plaque technique for recognizing individual antibody forming cells. In

C. A. Williams and M. W. Chase, Eds., *Methods in Immunology and Immunochemistry* vol. IV (Academic: New York, in press).

6.   Landy, M., Sanderson, R. P., and Jackson, A. L. Humoral and cellular aspects of the immune response to the somatic antigen of *Salmonella enteritidis. J. Exptl. Med. 122*, 483 (1965).

7.   Merchant, B. and Hraba, T. Lymphoid cells producing antibodies against simple haptens: Detection and enumeration. *Science 152*, 1378 (1966).

8.   Segre, D. and Segre, M. Hemolytic plaque formation by mouse spleen cells producing antibodies against rabbit immunoglobulin G. *J. Immunol. 99*, 867 (1967).

PASSIVE CUTANEOUS ANAPHYLAXIS

Passive cutaneous anaphylaxis (PCA) is a phenomenon in which an observable skin reaction can be produced in an animal by interaction of antigen and antibody. Classically, an antiserum is injected intradermally into the skin of a guinea pig. Antibodies become fixed to certain cells at the injected skin site. The corresponding antigen, together with an indicator dye, is injected intravenously. Upon reaching the injection site, the antigen reacts with the fixed antibodies. As a result of this reaction, pharmacologically-active substances, such as histamine, are released. These active substances increase the permeability of capillaries. As a result, the indicator dye becomes more concentrated in the area.

Generally two classes of antibodies are capable of fixing to the skin. These are termed homocytotropic and heterocytotropic. Homocytotropic antibodies can sensitize only the skin of the homologous species; heterocytotropic antibodies can sensitize only the skin of heterologous species. For example, in man, IgE antibodies (reaginic antibodies) are homocytotropic, since these antibodies fix only to the skin of man and other primates but do not fix to skin of other animals. The IgG antibodies of man are heterocytotropic, since they fix to the skin of guinea pigs but not to the skin of primates, including man. This complex subject is extensively reviewed by Block.

Materials

1.   Albino guinea pig, weighing 250-300 gm
2.   Monkey, *Macaca mulatta* or *irus*, weighing 6-8 lbs
3.   Antiserum: serum of individual sensitive to ragweed
4.   Antigen: ragweed extract
5.   Evans blue dye, 0.5% in saline solution

Method

1. PCA in guinea pig
    A. Shave the ventral side of a guinea pig with electric clippers. One can also use the skin of the back.

Note: *Do not irritate the skin. Handle the animal with care. Animals under stress are less reactive.*

    B. Inject intradermally, using a sharp 26 G needle, 0.1 ml of the proper dilution of the antiserum to be examined.

Note: *Do not pinch the skin.*

    C. Four to six hours later inject intravenously the antigen mixed with the Evans blue dye. The injection can be made in one of the foot veins. It is important to introduce no more than 2 ml of the dye-antigen mixture to avoid circulatory disturbances. The concentration of the antigen is very crucial in obtaining the optimal reaction.
    D. Read the reactions after 10 minutes. The reactions are graded according to the diameter and the intensity of the colored spots:

less than 5 mm	±
5-10 mm	+
10-15 mm	++
15-20 mm	+++
20 mm	++++

A strong positive reaction is easily observable on the external site of the skin. For more precise reading and when the reactions are weak, it is better to examine the internal side of the skin. For this purpose, the animal has to be sacrificed and the skin taken off.

2. PCA in monkey
    A. Tranquilize the animal using phencyclidine HCl 0.5-1 mg/kg.
    B. Remove the fur from the skin of the abdomen, thighs or cheeks by electric clippers.

Note: *Do not irritate the skin.*

    C. Inject intradermally, using a sharp 26 G needle, 0.05 ml of the proper dilution of the antiserum to be examined. The skin of the abdomen, thighs and cheeks are especially useful for passive sensitization.

Note: *Do not pinch the skin.*

D.   Inject intravenously the antigen mixed with the dye, 24-48 hours later. Approximately 5 ml of the antigen-dye may be injected. If preferred, one may inject the antigen locally (0.02 ml) into the same sites where the sera were injected and the dye alone (2-3 ml) afterwards intravenously.

E.   Read the reaction after 30 minutes. The reactions are graded according to the diameter and the intensity of the colored spots on the external side of the skin. (The arbitrary grading from ± to ++++ is used as described by guinea pig PCA.) When the antigen is injected locally, blue spots due to the trauma should not exceed 1-3 mm.

REFERENCES

1.   Block, K. J. The anaphylactic antibodies of mammals including man. In *Progress in Allergy*, vol. X (Karger: Basel, 1967), p. 84.
2.   Ishizaka, K., Ishizaka, T., and Arbesman, C. E. Introduction of passive cutaneous anaphylaxis in monkeys by human IgE antibody. *J. Aller. 39*, 254 (1967).
3.   Layton, L. L., Lee, S., and Dedds, F. Diagnosis of human allergy utilizing passive skin sensitization in the monkey *Macaca irus. Proc. Soc. Exptl. Biol. Med. 108*, 623 (1961).
4.   Ovary, Z. Immediate reactions in the skin of experimental animals provoked by antibody-antigen interaction. In *Progress in Allergy*, vol. V (Karger: Basel, 1958), p. 459.
5.   Rose, N. R., Kent, J. H., Reisman, R. E., and Arbesman, C. E. Demonstration of human reagin in the monkey. I. Passive sensitization of monkey skin with sera of untreated atopic patients. *J. Aller. 35*, 520 (1964).

IMMUNOCYTOADHERENCE (ROSETTE FORMATION)

This technique provides a method for quantitating the number of lymphoid cells that have specific receptors on their surface within a large lymphoid cell population. It is performed by mixing, in a liquid medium, spleen cells from an animal immunized with sheep erythrocytes with the immunizing antigen and then counting the number of lymphoid cells with adherent erythrocytes.

Materials

1.   Mice previously immunized with sheep erythrocytes
2.   Nonimmunized mice to serve as controls
3.   Eagle's minimum essential medium (MEM)
4.   Fetal calf serum (FCS)
5.   Sheep erythrocytes
6.   50-mesh-wire grid screen
7.   60 x 15 mm petri dishes
8.   Test tubes and capillary pipettes

Method

1.   Absorption of fetal calf serum
     A.   Wash sheep erythrocytes three times in phosphate-buffered saline (pH
          7.4).
     B.   To 1.0 ml of fetal calf serum, add 0.5 ml of washed packed sheep
          erythrocytes.
     C.   Incubate at 37°C for 30 minutes.
     D.   Centrifuge and take off serum.
2.   Preparation of incubation medium
     A.   Add 0.5 ml of absorbed FCS to 9.5 ml of MEM.
     B.   Add 0.2 ml of washed packed sheep erythrocytes to MEM.
3.   Preparation of spleen-cell suspension
     A.   Sacrifice a normal and an immunized mouse by cervical dislocation
          and remove their spleen.
     B.   Place each spleen on a 50-mesh-wire grid screen that is in a 60 x 15
          mm petri dish containing 10.0 ml of MEM.
     C.   Using the side of a scapel, force the spleen through the grid and into
          the MEM.
     D.   With a capillary pipette, aspirate the spleen-cell suspension several
          times to further disperse the cells and transfer the suspension to a
          large test tube.
     E.   After allowing the larger clumps to settle for 10 minutes, transfer the
          supernanant to a conical centrifuge tube and centrifuge for 5 minutes
          at 400 rpm.
     F.   Resuspend the cells in 5.0 ml of MEM-FCS, do a cell count with a
          hemocytometer, and prepare 1.0 ml of a cell suspension containing
          10^6 cells/0.1 ml.
4.   Performance of test
     A.   Place 0.9 ml of the sheep-cell suspension into each of two 12 x 75 mm

tubes.

B.   Add 0.1 ml of immune-spleen-cell suspension to one tube and 0.1 ml of normal-spleen-cell suspension to the other tube.

C.   Centrifuge the two tubes at 400-500 rpm for 15 minutes in a clinical centrifuge.

D.   With a capillary pipette, gently resuspend the cell pellet and place a small aliquot into a hemocytometer chamber.

E.   Count the number of lymphocytes with five or more adherent red cells that are present in the four large corner squares. Multiply this number by 2500 to give the number of positive cells per 10^6 spleen cells.

REFERENCES

1.   Biozzi, G., Stiffel, C., Mouton, D., Bouthillier, Y., and Decreusefond, C. A kinetic study of antibody producing cells in the spleen of mice immunized intravenously with sheep erythrocytes. *Immunol. 11*, 7 (1968).

2.   Brain, P., Gordon, J., and Willetts, A. Rosette formation by peripheral lymphocytes. *Clin. Exptl. Immunol. 6*, 681 (1970).

3.   Coombs, R. R. A., Gurner, B. W., Wilson, A. B., Holm, W. G., and Lindgren, B. Rosette-formation between human lymphocytes and sheep red cells not involving immunoglobulin receptors. *Int. Arch. Aller. 39*, 658 (1970).

4.   Moav, N. and Harris, T. N. Rosette formation in relation to active synthesis of antibody. *J. Immunol. 105*, 1501 (1970).

5.   Reyes, F. and Bach, J. F. Rosette-forming cells in the unimmunized mouse: Morphological studies with phase contrast and electron microscopy. *Cell. Immunol. 2*, 182 (1971).

6.   Zaalberg, O. B., van Der Meul, V. A., and van Twisk, J. M. Antibody production by isolated spleen cells: A study of the cluster and the plaque techniques. *J. Immunol. 100*, 451 (1968).

7.   Zaalberg, O. B., van Der Meul, V. A., and van Twisk, J. M. Antibody production by single spleen cells: A comparative study of the cluster and agar-plaque formation. *Nature 210*, 544 (1966).

IMMUNE CYTOTOXICITY

The cytotoxic test is based essentially on the interaction of antibody with living cells in the presence of complement. If antibodies (cytotoxins) combine with the target cells, complement is fixed and the cells are damaged. Although nucleated white blood cells have been used for the cytotoxic assay, the technique of cell culture offers a very convenient source of cells for the test.

It has also been demonstrated that "immune" or normal lymphocytes and macrophages when mixed with target cells in vitro may demonstrate cytolytic properties. Generally, the interaction between lymphocytes or macrophages and target cells does not require complement. Lambert and Hanes (1) were the first to demonstrate cytotoxins in sera of guinea pigs immunized with rat carcinoma, but the most widely used cytotoxic test was devised by Gorer and O'Gorman (6). For those who are interested in this topic, the review articles by Wissler and Flax (19), Winn (18), Waksman (14-15), and Wilson and Billingham (17) are recommended.

Cytotoxic reactions in vitro have been utilized in a variety of ways for the study of various biological systems. Of major interest is its use in histocompatibility testing for organ transplantation (13), the study of autoantibodies and sensitized lymphocytes in autoimmune diseases (8, 11), the detection of specific cellular antigens in establishing cell lines (1), and the study of the mechanism of homograft rejection and delayed hypersensitivity (12).

A variety of procedures and techniques have been developed for assessment and quantitation of cytotoxicity in vitro, depending on the particular system one is using. For general information these various techniques are listed below:

(1) microscopic examination of the target cells to detect morphological alterations (5, 7, 10),

(2) the ability of viable cells to exclude vital stains such as trypan blue, eosin Y, or erythrosin B (6),

(3) release of radioactive isotope from damaged target cells (16),

(4) the ability of target cells to form cones in agar after contact with antiserum or lymphoid cells (2),

(5) fluorochromasia (3),

(6) cytotoxic antiglobulin tests (4).

Materials

1. Sterile, heat-inactivated (56°C for 30 minutes), pre-immune serum from the animal to be immunized

2. Sterile, heat-inactivated antiserum against the particular target cells used

3. Complement (fresh frozen, sterile guinea pig serum)

Note: *Commercial complement cannot be used in cell cultures because preservatives added to lyophilized serum are toxic to tissue cells.*

4. Target cells. These may be either established cell lines maintained in the laboratory, primary cell cultures, or cell suspensions prepared from fresh tissue. In some experiments nucleated white cells of the reticuloendothelial system are used.
5. Tissue culture medium (e.g., Eagle's minimal essential medium, Medium 199, or Connaught Medical Research Laboratory Medium 1415)
6. Appropriate cell culture tubes. These may be Leighton tubes with coverslips, roller tubes, or plastic cell-culture petri dishes.
7. Sterile pipettes and glassware necessary for cell culture

Method

1. Cytotoxic test with serum and complement
    A. Prepare a consecutive series of dilutions of the antiserum in tissue culture (TC) medium.
    B. Prepare a similar series of dilutions of normal, pre-immune serum.
    C. Harvest the target cells by scraping with a "rubber policeman" into TC medium or with trypsin. Wash once with TC medium without serum. Make a cell count in a hemocytometer and dilute in TC medium to a predetermined cell concentration.
    D. Add 0.7 ml of the diluted target cell suspension to each of the culture tubes.
    E. Add 0.1 ml of the antiserum or normal-serum dilutions respectively to appropriate tubes.
    F. Add 0.2 ml of complement
    G. Mix the contents of each tube with gentle shaking and place in 37°C incubator. If Leighton tubes are being used, the coverslips must be straightened prior to incubation.
    H. Examine the cultures microscopically each day or, in some cases, after a few hours, for attachment and growth of the target cells.
    I. The test is read as the amount of cell growth in the tubes with antiserum as compared to the growth in the control tubes. The tubes are graded from − to ++++. A ++++ indicates no growth of the target cells and −, cell growth as in the control tubes.
2. Cytotoxic test with lymphoid cells on target cells
    A. Harvest target cells as indicated above. In some procedures the target cells are cultured in vitro for four to five hours or overnight to allow the cells to attach to the glass and spread.
    B. Aseptically remove lymph nodes and/or spleen from the immunized and normal (or control) animal, and place in TC medium. Trim the tissue free of all fat and connective tissue.

C. Prepare a cell suspension of the lymphoid cells. Tease the tissue apart in TC medium with needles, or mince the tissue cells with sterile blades and disperse the tissue cells by gentle agitation in a tissue grinder.

D. Allow the cell suspension to stand for 4-10 minutes in an upright centrifuge tube to permit debris and cell clumps to settle to the bottom.

E. Remove supernatant, wash the cells two or three times in TC medium (100 g for 10 minutes) and resuspend in TC medium.

F. Make a cell count in a hemocytometer and dilute cells to the appropriate concentration in TC medium. Usually several dilutions (e.g., twofold dilutions beginning with 5 million cells/ml) are prepared so that the effect of various numbers of lymphoid cells on the target cells can be determined.

G. If the target cells have been cultured to allow for their attachment, the culture medium is poured off and the cells washed by the addition of 1.0 ml of balanced saline solution.

H. Pour off the wash solution and add 1.0 ml of the various dilutions of the lymphoid cells to appropriate tubes.

I. Incubate the tubes at $37°C$ and read microscopically at 24, 48, and, in some instances, 72 hours for cell injury or inhibition of growth of the target cells.

J. Readings are taken and the tubes are scored from $-$ to $++++$ as indicated in section 1.

3. Release of radioactive chromium from damaged target cells

A. Harvest the target cells as previously described, wash and resuspend in a small volume (2-3) ml of PBS or TC medium.

B. Add 20-100 μc of $Na_2{}^{51}CrO_4$ (sodium chromate) to the target cell suspension and incubate at room temperature for 30-90 minutes.

C. Wash the target cells three times with large volumes of PBS or TC medium to remove all unbound chromium.

D. Dilute target cell suspension to appropriate concentration in TC medium.

Note: *The cell concentration is determined prior to the test by labeling a suspension of target cells and diluting them to various concentrations. These dilutions are then counted in a well-type γ scintillation counter to determine how effectively the cells labeled and how many are required in each tube to have sufficient radioactivity present.*

E. Remove 0.5 ml of the target cell suspension, place in a counting tube, and determine the amount of radioactivity incorporated by the cells by counting in a γ scintillation counter.

F. Add the appropriate volume of the labeled target cell suspension to each culture tube. Usually three to four replicates of each tube are prepared.

Note: *If the test is being done with serum and complement, 0.8 ml of the target cell suspension is added to each tube. Then 0.1 ml of the serum dilution is added to each tube and the tubes incubated at 37°C for 10 minutes. After incubation 0.2 ml of guinea pig complement (this may be commercial complement, as the cells are not going to be cultured for long periods of time) is added to each tube and the tubes replaced at 37°C. If the test is being done with lymphoid cells and target cells, 0.5 ml of each is added to each tube. The tubes are then incubated at 37°C.*

G. Remove at intervals of 30, 60, 90, and 120 minutes a single tube from each set and centrifuge at 500 g in the cold for 10 minutes. Remove 0.5 ml of the supernatant, place in a counting tube, and count in a γ scintillation counter to determine the amount of Cr-51 released into the medium by the target cells.

H. Express the results as the percent of total incorporated Cr-51 released into the medium.

REFERENCES

1. Bartholomew, W. R., Kite, J. H., and Rose, N. R. Antigens of mammalian cell cultures. II. The nature and cellular location of the cytotoxinogen in established cell lines. *Lab. Invest. 17*, 527 (1967).
2. Brunner, K. T., Mauel, J., and Schindler, R. In vitro studies of cell-bound immunity, cloning assay of the cytotoxic action of sensitized lymphoid cells on allogeneic target cells. *Immunol. 11*, 499 (1966).
3. Celada, F. and Rotman, B. A fluorochromatic test for immunotoxicity against tumor cells and leukocytes in agarose plates. *Proc. Nat. Acad. Sci. 57*, 630 (1967).
4. Fass, L. and Herberman, R. B. A cytotoxic antiglobulin technique for assay of antibodies to histocompatibility antigens. *J. Immunol. 102*, 140 (1969).
5. Goldberg, B. and Green, H. The cytotoxic action of immune gamma globulin and complement on Krebs ascites tumor cells. I. Ultrastructural studies. *J. Exptl. Med. 109*, 505 (1959).

6.   Gorer, P. and O'Gorman, P. The cytotoxic activity of isoantibodies in mice. *Trans. Bull. 3*, 142 (1956).

7.   Green, H., Fleischer, R. A., Barrow, P., and Goldberg, B. The cytotoxic action of immune gamma globulin and complement on Krebs ascites tumor cells. II. Chemical studies. *J. Exptl. Med. 109*, 511 (1959).

8.   Kite, J. H., Rose, N. R., Kano, K., and Witebsky, E. Cytotoxicity of human thyroid autoantibodies. *Ann. N. Y. Acad. Sci. 124*, 626 (1965).

9.   Lambert, R. A. and Hanes, F. M. The cultivation of tissue in vitro as a method for the study of cytotoxins. *J. Exptl. Med. 14*, 453 (1911).

10.   Miller, D. G. and Hsu, T. C. The action of cytotoxic antisera on the HeLa strain of human carcinoma. *Cancer Res. 16*, 306 (1955).

11.   Perlmann, P. and Broberger, O. In vitro studies of ulcerative colitis. II. Cytotoxic action of white blood cells from patients on human fetal colon cells. *J. Exptl. Med. 117*, 705 (1963).

12.   Ruddle, N. H. and Waksman, B. H. Cytotoxicity mediated by soluble antigen and lymphocytes in delayed hypersensitivity. I, II, and III. *J. Exptl. Med. 128*, 1237 (1968).

13.   von Rood, J. J. and Eernisse, J. G. The detection of transplantation antigens in leukocytes. *Seminars in Hematol. 5*, 187 (1968).

14.   Waksman, B. H. *Progress in Allergy 5*, 349 (1958).

15.   ——————. The toxic effects of the antigen-antibody reaction on the cells of hypersensitive reactors. In H. S. Lawrence, Ed. *Cellular and Humoral Aspects for the Hypersensitive States* (Paul B. Hoeber, Harper & Bros.: New York, 1959), p. 123.

16.   Wigsell, H. Quantitative titrations of mouse H-2 antibodies using Cr^{51}-labelled target cells. *Transplantation 3*, 423 (1965).

17.   Wilson, D. B. and Billingham, R. E. Lymphocytes and transplantation immunity. *Adv. in Immunol. 7*, 189 (1967).

18.   Winn, H. J. The immune response and homograft rejection. *Nat. Cancer Inst. Monogr. 2*, 113 (1960).

19.   Wissler, R. W. and Flax, M. A. Cytotoxic effects of antitumor serum. *Ann. N. Y. Acad. Sci. 69*, 773 (1957).

Chapter 9

PREPARATIVE PROCEDURES

C. J. van Oss

GEL FILTRATION

Gel filtration, or molecular sieve chromatography, is a preparative method for
the separation of proteins according to size. A column is used in which dextran
gel beads suspended in buffer have been allowed to settle. The pore size of the
gel granules is chosen in such a manner that the larger proteins that are to be
separated cannot penetrate them but go around them, while the smaller proteins
that can penetrate them will perforce do so and thus will follow a much longer
path.

In a column the nonpenetrant molecules remain in the interstices and
appear in the effluent following an elution volume equal to the void volume of
the column. Smaller molecules appear after a larger volume of eluant has passed,
depending on their degree of penetration. When a volume equal to the total
solvent volume of the bed has been reached, all solutes have been eluted from
the column, except when adsorption has occurred.

Materials

The dextran gel beads most generally used are those of Pharmacia in Sweden,
named Sephadex. The different grades available are called G-200, G-75, G-50,
and G-25. These figures indicate that the pores of these gel beads will totally
exclude proteins of a molecular weight of, respectively, 200,000, 75,000,
50,000, and 25,000. Typical applications of Sephadex G-100 or G-200 are the
fractionation and purification of plasma proteins, enzymes, and also nonprotein-
aceous materials such as polysaccharides and nucleic acids. The sample may be
flushed through the column using any one of several solutions (e.g., TRIS-HCl
[0.1 M + 0.2 M NaCl, pH 8.0], 0.9% NaCl, buffered saline, or 1.0M acetic acid
[when H and L chains of immunoglobulins are to be separated]).

175

Method

1. Swelling of gel beads: Before being poured into a column, Sephadex G-100 or G-200 should be allowed to swell in an excess of the buffer to be used. A small amount of fine particles often gives the supernatant a turbid appearance. These can be removed by suction. The swelling of the gel particles takes one to three days. The swelling procedure can be shortened by boiling the Sephadex.
2. Pouring the column
    A. The column is filled one-third full with the buffer of choice.
    B. A thick slurry of (for instance) G-200 is added. The gel particles are allowed to settle until a layer (about 10 cm) has formed.
    C. The outlet is then opened, and as the supernatant (above the gel bed) clears, it can be carefully removed and more Sephadex added until the column is filled to about 5 cm from the top.
    D. When pouring is finished, the column is connected to the buffer reservoir. The bed is stabilized by washing overnight.
3. Introduction of the sample
    A. The liquid above the bed is carefully removed.
    B. The sample is slowly layered on the surface of the Sephadex, taking care that the bed surface is not disturbed.
    C. The bottom outlet is opened after the sample has been layered on the bed.
    D. The sample must completely enter the Sephadex.
    E. Buffer is added up to the top of the column and connected with the buffer reservoir. The airtight system should have approximately 6-12 cm of hydrostatic pressure (as judged by the distance from the column bottom to the buffer surface in the reservoir).
    F. The flow rate must be adjusted to approximately 4-6 ml/cm^2/h.
4. Fraction collection
    A. Fractions are usually collected in 4-5-ml portions.
    B. The protein concentration of the fractions is usually determined by reading their OD in a spectrophotometer at 280 nm (ultraviolet).
    C. Finally, the curve of protein concentration versus tube number is plotted on graph paper, in order to visualize the whereabouts of the various fractions obtained. Serum proteins are generally collected in the order: macroglobulins, globulins, albumin.

REFERENCES

1. Determann, H. *Gel Chromatography* (Springer: New York, 1968).

2.   Porath, T. Cross-linked dextrans as molecular sieves. *Adv. Prot. Chem. 17*, 209 (1962).

ION-EXCHANGE CHROMATOGRAPHY

Ion-exchange chromatography involves the electrostatic binding of proteins onto an electrically charged cellulose derivative suspended in buffer and packed into a column. Elution (desorption) is accomplished by changing the pH of buffer passing through the column, thus affecting the charge of the protein molecules (and also, in some cases, the charge on the adsorbent). At the same time, the molarity of the buffer is increased. thereby facilitating the dissociation of electrostatic linkages between the proteins and the adsorbent.

Conditions for chromatography are selected to take advantage of net charge differences between serum proteins and to assure a net charge on the resin opposite that of the proteins. By a gradual increase in salt concentration, with or without a fall in pH, proteins are eluted in order of increasing numbers of charged groups bound to the resin. The behavior of very large molecules, such as IgM, is at variance with this description because in such instances adsorption due to van der Waal's forces plays a larger role than adsorption due to electrostatic forces.

Both anion and cation exchange resins are available. Diethyl amino ethyl (DEAE) cellulose is used as an anion exchanger and carboxymethyl (CM) cellulose as cation exchanger.

Materials

1.   DEAE cellulose. DEAE cellulose may be obtained in floc or powder form.
2.   0.1N NaOH
3.   Buffers:

	0.0175M	pH 6.3	$Na_2 HPO_4$
	0.04M	pH 5.9	$Na_2 HPO_4$
	0.10M	pH 5.8	$Na_2 HPO_4$
	0.40M	pH 5.2	$Na_2 HPO_4$
	0.40M	pH 4.4	$Na_2 HPO_4$ + 2M NaCl

4.   Column to hold 10 x 37 cm resin bed
5.   Fraction collector
6.   Serum

Method

1.   Suspend 15 g of DEAE cellulose in 0.1N sodium hydroxide and allow to

remain overnight.

2. The next day filter it under gentle suction on a Büchner funnel, and wash alternately with distilled water and 0.1N sodium hydroxide for a total of three cycles.

3. After the last 0.1N sodium hydroxide wash, the DEAE is washed three times more with distilled water and is then suspended in starting buffer, 0.0175M, pH 6.3 sodium phosphate. It is then washed with this buffer until the effluent arrives at this pH.

4. The column outlet is closed, and the cellulose suspension is poured in. As the cellulose accumulates on the bottom, the outlet is opened and more suspension is poured in until the entire amount has been added.

5. The column is packed by flushing several volumes of starting buffer through it from a buffer reservoir.

6. Next, 30 ml of serum that has been dialyzed versus the starting buffer is carefully layered on top of the resin bed after the buffer layer is removed. (Dialyzed serum should be centrifuged to remove insoluble material.)

7. Open the outlet after the sample has passed into the cellulose, carefully fill to the top with buffer, and reconnect the buffer reservoir.

8. Collect 10-ml fractions. The effluent is monitored by reading the optical density of each fraction in a spectrophotometer at 280 nm and preparing a plot of optical density versus fraction number. Once a peak has been obtained and readings have dropped and leveled off, the next buffer (0.04M, pH 5.9) is passed through the column, and so on, until all the fractions have been eluted. In this way five major fractions of serum may be obtained:

0.0175M	pH 6.3:IgG
0.04M	pH 5.9:β globulins
0.10M	pH 5.8:albumin
0.40M	pH 5.2:α globulins
0.40M	pH 4.4 + 2M NaCl:IgM

Note: *For the isolation of a single protein from a mixture, it is not always necessary to use a column. The "batch method," described by Stanworth (2) has proven quite useful for the isolation of human IgG from whole serum. In this method DEAE cellulose is washed as described above (steps 1-3) and is then equilibrated with a 0.01M phosphate buffer of pH 7.5 (containing 0.015M sodium chloride). Then, 2.5 ml of serum (dialyzed against the same buffer) is added to 30 g (moist) of the above DEAE cellulose. The mixture is then kept at 4°C for five hours. The DEAE cellulose is centrifuged in a refrigerated centrifuge. The supernatant thus obtained contains virtually pure IgG.*

REFERENCES

1. Sober, H. A. and Peterson, E. A. Protein chromatography on ion exchange cellulose. *Federation Proc. 17*, 1116 (1958).
2. Stanworth, D.R. A rapid method of preparing pure serum gamma-globulin. *Nature 188*, 156 (1960).

STARCH BLOCK ELECTROPHORESIS

Starch block electrophoresis is the simplest preparative electrophoretic method, permitting the fractionation of up to 10 ml blood serum, in a batch process, which lasts about 24 hours.

Materials

1. Potato starch (Fisher S-514, unhydrolyzed)
2. Barbital buffer, $\Gamma/2 = 0.05$, pH 8.6 (barbital, 104 g; 10N NaOH, 48 ml; water 24 l)
3. Electrophoresis chamber and tray (35.5 x 10 x 1 cm)
4. Power supply (capable of at least 300 V and 50 mA)
5. Paper wicks, 9 x 10 cm cut from Whatman no. 3MM paper

Method

1. To 300 g of Fisher potato starch is added 270 ml of barbital buffer, pH 8.6, ionic strength 0.05. When the starch and buffer are of a uniform consistency, the mixture is poured into a plastic mold which is 35.5 cm by 10 cm Fig. 9.1.) The open ends of the mold or block are closed by means of fitted plastic end pieces, which are held tightly in place by means of a rubber band encircling the whole block. A piece of Whatman filter paper (no. 3MM) is cut so that it covers the bottom 2.5 cm of each end of the block and about 8 cm is folded and hanging over the endpieces. A similar piece is placed on the top of the ends of the starch after it has been poured into the block. These pieces help to produce uniform electrical conduction. The starch is air-dried at room temperature until it seems quite hard and slightly powdery. This development can be accelerated by placing pieces of filter paper over the entire top of the starch to absorb the excess moisture. When the starch is adequately dried, the top layer is scraped off until it is level and smooth.
2. A well is then cut into the starch about 15 cm from the cathode end of the

block. This well is approximately 1 x 7 cm and is cut perpendicular to the long axis of the block. It is filled with a mixture of about 5 ml of normal human serum and enough dry potato starch to enable it to be poured as a thickened liquid. In this manner the well can be completely filled and the extract will not seep into the surrounding starch block. The top of the block is then entirely covered with a glass plate. The plastic endpieces are removed, leaving only the filter-paper pieces, which extend from the bottom of the mold to cover the ends of the starch block.

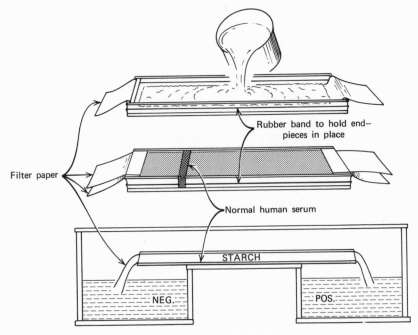

Fig. 9.1.

3. The block is then placed in the electrophoresis chamber (Fig. 9.1). The chamber is filled with about 2 l of barbital buffer, pH 8.6, ionic strength of 0.05. The filter-paper strips dip into the buffer. The electrodes are connected to a Spinco Duostat power supply. The run takes place in a cold room (4°C) at a constant setting of 250 V and a current with ranges from 10-20mA. The latter seems to vary with the degree of dryness of the block at the time of preparation. The electrophoresis time is about 24 hours.

4. At the end of the run the glass plate is slid off and the starch is cut into 1-cm-wide segments, numbered from the cathode glass end of the

block. Each segment is placed into a sintered (coarse) glass funnel resting in a 50-ml polypropylene centrifuge tube. They are spun at room temperature in a Sorvall SP/X centrifuge at about 3000 rpm for about five minutes, and these first eluates are used for protein determination. These eluates are generally about 1 ml in volume and clear. Next 2 ml of the same barbital buffer are added to the powdery starch that remains in the funnel, and after spinning under the same conditions, this second eluate is placed in other test tubes to be combined with the first group, after the latter is analyzed for protein concentration. Protein concentration is estimated by the biuret method. In general, 0.05 ml of sample is mixed with 2.00 ml of biuret reagent and, after color development, is read in a spectrophotometer at a wavelength of 540 nm. From these readings, a graph of optical density versus fraction number may be prepared.

REFERENCES

1. Bloemendal, H. *Zone Electrophoresis in Blocks and Columns* (Elsevier: New York, 1963).
2. Kunkel, H. and Trautman, R. Zone electrophoresis in various types of supporting media. In M. Bier, Ed., *Electrophoresis* (Academic: New York, 1959).
3. Shulman, S., Rapp, D., Bronson, P., and Arbesman, C. E. Immunologic studies of caddis fly. II. Isolation of the allergic fraction of caddis fly extract. *J. Aller. 33*, 438 (1962).

SDS-POLYACRYLAMIDE GEL ELECTROPHORESIS

Electrophoresis in dense gels is a method that has been used for a long time. It separates proteins according to size as well as according to charge. The one drawback of the method is that it is impossible to determine, when any separation is done, whether separation was caused by a difference in size, a difference in charge, or a combination of both. Recently, however, it has been made possible by the admixture of sodium dodecyl sulfate (SDS) to the proteins, which lends them a uniform strong negative charge, to separate by electrophoresis in a dense gel all proteins according to their size only (because when the electric charge is the same for all proteins, differences in mobility can now only be caused by differences in size).

Materials and Methods

Gels are usually prepared from a mixture of acrylamide monomer (95 parts) and methylene-bis-acrylamide cross linkage agent (5 parts) in concentration of 4-10% (or higher), although the proportions are changed for the higher concentrations. Electrophoresis is commonly carried out in 7.5% gels at a pH of 8-9. Details of such experiments are best obtained from the manufacturer of the apparatus being used.

One may use a Beckman Microzone accessory, which permits flat-bed horizontal electrophoresis, as contrasted to the frequently seen individual gel-tube vertical electrophoresis. The flat-bed arrangement is advantageous when mobility comparisons are to be made, because it permits the running of several samples in the same gel under precisely the same operating conditions.

In this experiment, a 7.5% gel prepared in pH 8.8, 0.065M Tris-glycine buffer with an SDS concentration of 0.10%, has been used for the separation of various proteins after they have been incubated at 37°C for two hours in 1% SDS. Migration is dependent on size alone in such a system. A plot of log molecular weight versus relative mobility (using some low-molecular-weight protein as a standard) reveals a sigmoidal-shaped curve that has a rather large linear section in the 15,000-30,000 molecular weight range. With the use of suitable standards, it is possible to contruct a calibration curve from which, knowing the relative mobility of an unknown, the molecular weight may be ascertained to within 5-6% of its real value.

An innovative use of this method combines immunodiffusion with polyacrylamide-SDS gel electrophoresis, to permit the immunochemical identification of a given substance as well as the molecular weight. This method is advantageous in a system of molecular heterogeneity Where a specific antiserum permits the localization of the band of interest. Essentially, the method parallels standard immunoelectrophoresis with the two major differences being that the proteins to be evaluated are treated with SDS and that the electrophoresis is carried out in polyacrylamide-SDS gels, followed by diffusion in agar.

REFERENCES

1.   *Beckman Model 113 Acrylamide Gel Accessory Instruction Manual, RM-TB-015A* (Spinco Division of Beckman Instruments Inc.: Palo Alto, Calif., May 1970).
2.   Dubert, J. M., Hermier, B., and Babinet, C. Essai de caractérisation immunochemie des fractions présentes dans une préparation de RNA poly-

mérase d'*E. coli. Biochimie 53*, 185 (1971).

3.   Dunker, A. K. and Ruechkert, R. R. Observation on molecular weight determinations of polyacrylamide gel. *J. Biol. Chem. 244*, 5074 (1969).

4.   Shapiro, A. L., Vinuela, E., and Maizel, J. V. Molecular weight estimation of polypeptide chains by electrophoresis in SDS-polyacrylamide gels. *Biochem. Biophys. Res. Commun. 28*, 815 (1967).

ULTRAFILTRATION

Since the discovery in the early 1960's of the possibility of making ultrafiltration membranes with an ultrathin top skin (which is the actual ultrafiltrating barrier) on top of a much more porous layer of conventional thicknesses, very high-flux protein-stopping membranes have become feasible. With commercially available apparatus and with commercially available membranes or with membranes made in the laboratory, it is now possible to concentrate 500 ml of a dilute protein solution more than 300 times in the course of one afternoon, without incurring any protein denaturation.

Materials

1.   Ultrafilters. The only usable ultrafilters commercially available are made by the Amicon Corporation (Lexington, Mass.) Besides an ultrafilter, a source of compressed nitrogen must be available, with a pressure regulator.

2.   Membranes. Protein-stopping membranes are very easily made in the laboratory in the following way: Cellulose diacetate (39.8% acetate, ASTM viscosity 3, Eastman no. 4644; to be kept in a vacuum desiccator) is used as the membrane material. Under constant stirring with a pestle, 25 g of this are slowly added to 75 ml of acetone and 50 ml of formamide in a mortar of at least 130-mm diameter opening. Stirring is continued until all lumps are dissolved. The mixture is then poured into a 500-ml filtering flask and placed in a waterbath kept at 50-55°C. About 40 cm Hg vacuum is applied to the flask, until all bubbles (caused by stirring) have disappeared. Approximately 15 ml of the mixture is then poured in a ribbon across the short side of a 17 x 25 cm glass plate (along the two long edges of which two 0.15-0.30 mm thick metal runners are clamped: the thinner the runners, the thinner the membrane and the higher the flux). The mixture is then quickly and evenly spread over the glass plate, with the help of a 15-cm-long glass test tube, by drawing the tube in one smooth horizontal motion along the runners. An excess of about two-thirds of the applied mixture is swept off the glass plate and should be discarded. As quickly as possible,

the glass plate with the spread-out mixture must be submerged in an ice-water bath (a 20 x 30 cm tray, filled with tap water and an abundance of ice cubes can be used) and kept there for one hour, after which the membrane can be lifted from the plate. The almost instantaneous coagulation of the upper surface of the mixture, upon its immersion in cold water, causes the membrane to be provided with a very thin skin that is denser than the rest of the membrane structure. This is the actual protein-stopping skin, so that care must be taken always to use the membrane with the side up that was away from the glass plate when it was formed. For immediate and even future use, the membrane is best kept in cold (tap) water. For longer conservation, up to 20% ethanol may be added to the water, to avoid spoilage. Sheets of membrane, prepared as described above, yield two circular membranes of 7.5-cm diameter, plus another two or three membranes of 4.7-cm diameter, at a total cost of a few dimes. In order not to lose sight of the "skinned" side of the membrane, the best practice is to cut circular membranes out of the larger sheet only as and when needed and to mark the edge of the larger sheets in some asymmetrical fashion (for instance, with the help of a card perforator).

Method

For the prevention of concentration polarization or clogging of the membrane's pores by a buildup of very high protein concentrations localized on top of the membrane, continuous stirring of the protein solution above the membrane is a condition sine qua non for any ultrafiltration involving more than a few milliliters of protein solution. With most skinned membranes the optimal pressure is 30 lb/in.^{2} when ultrafiltering concentrated protein solutions (1% protein and more), but at lower protein concentrations somewhat higher pressures can be used, in order to obtain faster ultrafiltration. The most inert source of pressure is compressed nitrogen, from a high-pressure nitrogen bottle provided with a 1-100-lb/in.^{2} pressure regulating valve and 1-100-lb/in.^{2} and 1-3000-lb/in.^{2} gauges. With the consecutive use of the Diaflo 400 and 50 cells (Amicon Co.), 400 ml of a dilute protein solution can first be reduced to about 30-40 ml in the large cell, within about two hours. The total membrane surface of that cell is too large, however, to concentrate the solution much further than down to about 30-40 ml, because at that point the height of the liquid column has become too low for the stirrer to have any effect. But the last 30-40 ml can easily be further reduced to as little as 1 ml in the second, smaller cell, in about one hour. The last few milliliters will no longer be stirred, but at the end of the process, this will create no unacceptable losses. The final concentrate can be poured out, aspirated with a pipette, or, after piercing the membrane with a needle, forced out of the ultrafilter with the help of compressed nitrogen. Thus, 400 ml of a dilute protein solution can be concentrated to 1 ml in about three hours.

There now also exists a thin anisotropic membrane made of a mixture of cellulose nitrate and cellulose acetate that allows the removal of all IgM from a portion of a serum sample in about 20 minutes with the help of either a centrifuge-tube ultrafilter and a tabletop centrifuge or a small-pressure-ultrafilter cell.

The membrane is made as follows: A 500-ml Sorvall Omnimixer (Ivan Sorvall, Norwalk, Conn.) chamber is filled with 50 ml glacial acetic acid and 40 ml acetone. To this mixture is added 15 g cellulose nitrate (30% ethanol, viscosity 16.2, grade DHB 14 E, Du Pont). The whole is then mixed in the Omnimixer, and once the mixture is uniform, 15 g cellulose diacetate (39.8% acetate, ASTM viscosity 3, Eastman no. 4644) and 40 ml formamide are added to the chamber. Mixing is resumed until the mixture is uniform. (If no mixer is available, the ingredients can be put into a stoppered flask and allowed to dissolve overnight.) Vacuum (approximately 40 cm Hg) is then applied to the flask until all air bubbles have disappeared. Approximately 15 ml of the mixture is then poured in a ribbon across the short side of a 17 x 25 cm stainless-steel plate, along the two long edges of which two 0.25-mm-thick metal runners are clamped. (Contrary to an earlier described membrane, glass plates cannot be used for casting this membrane because of an excessive stickiness of the above described material to glass; stainless steel does not have that drawback.) The mixture is then spread quickly and evenly over the stainless-steel plate with the help of a 15-cm-long glass test tube, by drawing the tube in one smooth horizontal movement along the runners. An excess of about two-thirds of the applied mixture is swept off the plate and discarded. Once drawn, the membrane is "super-skinned" with the aid of an air blast (at 20°C) provided by a hair dryer (model 202 Oster, Milwaukee, Wis.), held 15 cm above the plate for 60 seconds, after which the plate is immersed in an ice-water bath, in which it remains for at least one hour prior to use. The membrane can then be lifted from the plate. The strong evaporation of solvent at the upper surface of the viscous mixture, coupled with the almost instantaneous coagulation of that top surface upon its immersion in cold water, provides the membrane with a very thin skin that is denser than the rest of the membrane structure. This is the actual protein-retaining skin, and care must be taken always to use the membrane with the side up that was away from the metal plate when it was formed. For immediate and even for future use, the membrane is best kept in cold (tap) water. In order not to lose sight of the skinned side of the membrane, the best practice is to cut circular membranes out of the larger sheet only as needed and to mark the edge of the larger sheet in some asymmetrical fashion. As measured by scanning electron microscopy, the actual "skin" is about 0.3 μ thick. The flow rate of the membrane is about 150 ml/h/100 cm^2/10 lb/in.^{2} for 1% protein, and 60 ml/h when ultrafiltering whole serum. The optimal pressure is 10 lb/in.^{2}, but pressures up to 20 lb/in.^{2} may be used; at higher pressures than that, leakage may occur. It is rarely feasible in practice to obtain more than 10-20% of the protein in the ultrafiltrate, because the protein concentration of the ultrafiltrate is significantly lower than that of the serum being ultrafiltered. (For example, when whole serum with 7.5% protein is ultrafiltered, the ultrafiltrate will contain 1.5-2.1% protein.) But the important aspect is that the ultrafiltrate will be devoid of macroglobulins, while albumin and the 7 S globulins are present in close to normal proportions.

REFERENCES

1. van Oss, C. J., McConnell, C. R., Tompkins, R. K., and Bronson, P. M. A membrane for the rapid concentration of dilute protein samples in an ultrafilter. *Clin. Chem. 15*, 699 (1969).
2. van Oss, C. J. and Bronson, P. M. Characteristics of a protein concentrating anisotropic cellulose acetate membrane. *Separation Sci. 5*, 63 (1970).
3. ——————. Separation of blood serum proteins by ultrafiltration. In J. E. Flinn, Ed., *Membrane Science and Technology*, (proceedings of a symposium held at Battelle Memorial Inst., Columbus, Ohio, Oct. 20-21, 1969; Plenum: New York, 1970).
4. ——————. Removal of IgM from serum by ultrafiltration. *Analyt. Biochem. 36*, 464 (1970).

ZONE ULTRACENTRIFUGATION

For the preparative separation of protein mixtures into several fractions of different molecular weights by ultracentrifugation only zone centrifugation is suitable. For reasons of stability, zone ultracentrifugation can only be done on liquid columns of a continuously increasing (from meniscus to bottom) density. In other words, the mixture to be separated has to be layered on top of a preexisting density gradient. For that reason, this method is also sometimes called density-gradient ultracentrifugation. Batchwise separations are done in rotors that contain separate tubes. Generally, in order to avoid remixing after stopping the rotor, these tubes are held in "swinging buckets." Continuous separations are done in density-gradients contained in "zonal rotors." Here only the batch method, with density gradients in tubes in swinging-bucket rotors, will be treated.

Materials

1. A Model L Spinco preparative ultracentrifuge
2. An SW39 or 50 rotor
3. Three cellulose nitrate tubes, 0.5 x 2 in.
4. 10% sucrose in saline solution
5. 40% sucrose in saline solution
6. A 2-ml syringe
7. 3 ml of 50% serum in saline

Method

1. Each of three cellulose nitrate tubes is partially filled with 2 ml of 10% sucrose in saline. Then, with the help of a syringe, 2 ml of the 40% sucrose (also dissolved in saline) is injected under the 10% sucrose layer. The tubes are then allowed to stand undisturbed for 24 hours at 4°C, allowing an optimal density gradient to form, by simple molecular diffusion.
2. Once the gradient is formed, 1 ml of the 50% diluted serum is layered on top of each of the gradients. The tubes are then put into the swinging-bucket rotor and spun at 39,000 rpm for 18 hours.
3. The rotor is then (slowly) stopped, and from each tube the fractions are collected by piercing their bottoms with an injection needle and by allowing the drops, five at a time, to fall into successive collection tubes.
4. The protein concentration of the fractions is then determined by reading their optical density in a spectrophotometer at 280 mμ. The curve of optical density versus fraction number can then be plotted, in order to visualize the whereabouts of the fractions that have been obtained. With normal serum the macroglobulins are in the lower quarter, the other globulins in the middle, and albumin in the upper third of the tube.

REFERENCES

1. Dudworth, D. W. Calibration curves for density-gradient columns. *J. Sci. Instrum. 39*, 377 (1962).
2. Kunkel, H. G. Macroglobulins and high molecular weight antibodies. In F. W. Putnam, Ed., *The Plasma Proteins*, vol. I (Academic: New York, 1960).

IMMUNOADSORBENTS

Efforts are made to isolate antibodies in a pure state from a serum or other protein mixture. Campbell, Luescher, and Lerman were the first who used insoluble antigens for isolation of antibodies. The isolation of the antibodies involves:

(1) insolubilization of the antigen;

(2) adsorption of the specific antibodies by the insoluble antigen;

(3) elution of the antibodies from the antigen.

Insolubilization of the antigens may be achieved either by polymerizing the antigens themselves to make them insoluble, or by coupling the antigens to insoluble carriers such as cellulose derivatives or other polymers.

Immunoadsorbents are also used for the radioimmunoassay of minute amounts of antigens.

Materials

1. Preparation of rabbit serum albumin (RSA) polymer
    A. S-acetylmercaptosuccinylation
        (1) Dissolve RSA 3 g (0.046 m moles) in 75 ml borate buffer, pH 8.0, and stir under N_2 stream.
        (2) Add S-acetylmercaptosuccinic anhydride 221 mg (1.27 m moles) in small portions maintaining pH at 8.0 with M-NaOH over one hour.
        (3) Dialyze overnight against cold saline buffered at pH 8.0 (S-AMS-RSA).
    B. Deacetylation
        (1) Stir S-AMS-RSA under N_2 stream at room temperature.
        (2) Add N-NaOH to raise pH to 11.5.
        (3) Maintain pH 11.5 with N-NaOH for 45-60 minutes.
    C. Polymerization
        (1) Add N-HCl to lower the pH to 8.0.
        (2) Add 0.92 ml MAPO (4.6 m moles) (Tris 1-2-methyl, aziridinyl, phosphine oxide. Lederle Laboratories, Pearl River, N.Y.).
        (3) Add N-HCl to lower the pH to 4.0 (heavy precipitate is formed).
        (4) Stir for three hours, maintaining pH 4.0 with N-HCl. N_2 stream is used until the completion of this step.
        (5) Continue stirring overnight in the cold.
    D. Washing
        (1) Centrifuge the reaction mixture at 2500 rpm for 10 minutes. Discard supernatant.
        (2) Wash precipitate twice with saline.
        (3) Wash precipitate three times with 500 ml of 1M propionic acid containing 0.8% NaCl or 0.1M glycine-HCl buffer, pH 2.5, in the

cold.

(4) Suspend washed precipitate in saline to form a thick slurry.

(5) Pour the slurry into 500 ml 0.2M borate buffer, pH 8.0, under stirring and adjust pH to 8.0 with NaOH (precipitate swells).

(6) Centrifuge and discard the supernatant.

(7) Disperse precipitate with a loosely fitted glass homogenizer.

(8) Wash precipitate repeatedly until OD_{280} of the washing fluids is lower than 0.05.

(9) Suspend washed precipitate in borate buffer, pH 8.0.

(10) Store the RSA polymer in a refrigerator.

(11) The polymer content of a suspension can be measured by Lowry's method (Folin) with the product solubilized by digestion with pronase at pH 8.0, or by heating briefly with 0.5N NaOH.

2. Coupling of p-azobenzenearsonate (Rp) groups to RSA polymer

A. Take RSA-polymer suspension containing 150 mg polymer (2.2 μ moles) and centrifuge.

B. Suspend polymer in 15 ml borate buffer, pH 9.0, cool in ice.

C. Cool 2.5 ml 0.02M p-arsanilic acid in 0.05N HCl (50 μ moles) in ice. While stirring, add 0.1M $NaHO_2$ drop by drop until slight excess. About 0.5 ml is required. KI starch paper is used to detect excess NO_2.

D. Stir polymer suspension in ice. Add the above solution drop by drop. Stir the mixture for three hours in ice.

E. Centrifuge and wash the precipitate repeatedly with borate buffer, pH 8.0, until the supernatant fluid is colorless.

F. Suspend precipitate (Rp-RSA-polymer) in borate buffer, pH 8.0. Number of Rp-groups coupled to RSA polymer can be measured spectrophotometrically on the product solubilized by digestion with pronase.

3. Coupling of bovine serum albumin (BSA) to RSA polymer

A. Bis-diazodized benzidine (BDB). Cool 5 ml of benzidine dihydrochloride solution (0.2M in 0.1N HCl) and 10 ml $NaHO_2$ (0.04M) in ice. Add $NaNO_2$ drop by drop to benzidine until the reaction remains positive with starch-KI paper (moistened with 1N HCl) for 15 minutes after last addition of $NaNO_2$. About 5 ml of $NaNO_2$ is required.

B. Suspend 200 mg of prewashed RSA polymer in 5 ml of 0.2M phosphate buffer, pH 7.5, cool in ice, and under good stirring, mix quickly with 3.1 ml of BDB (check pH). After 1-2 minutes, add 10 ml of ice-cold BSA solution (20-50 mg/ml, pH 7.5 buffer) very rapidly (check pH).

C.   Stir on ice for two hours and then in the coldroom overnight; pH should be over 7 throughout the procedure.

D.   Wash precipitate with glycine-HCl buffer, pH 2.4, in cold and then with borate buffer, pH 8.0.

4.   Polymerization of γ globulin with glutaraldehyde reagents

A.   γ-globulin solution. 10 mg/ml in 0.1M acetate buffer, pH 4.9.

B.   Glutaraldehyde. 25% (2.5M) aqueous solution (Eastman Kodak) or 50% (5M) aqueous solution (Fisher Sci.).

C.   Cellulose powder. Munktell no. 400 is suitable for both column and batch use.

Methods

1.   Take 100 ml of γ-globulin solution (1 g) in a 400 ml beaker and add 2 g cellulose powder under stirring. (More cellulose may be added to expand the volume of absorbent).

2.   Add 1.0 ml 2.5M glutaraldehyde (use propipette) and 10 g Na_2SO_4 powder in small proportions. Stir the mixture continuously.

3.   From time to time, take a small portion of the mixture, dilute with four volumes of 0.1M Tris-HCl, pH 8.0, and centrifuge. Take the supernatant and add trichloracetic acid to a final concentration of 5% to test the presence of soluble protein. Normally, polymerization is almost complete in 60 minutes when IgG or IgM is used. With other proteins such as IgA or Bence-Jones proteins, polymerization may not be evident in 60 minutes. In such a case, add 1 ml more of 25% glutaraldehyde and continue the reaction. Addition of more Na_2SO_4 also accelerates the polymerization.

4.   After 120 minutes (when polymerization is complete), filter the mixture with a sintered glass filter (Medium), wash the filter cake once with acetate buffer, and resuspend in 50 ml acetate buffer.

5.   Add 5 g glycine and stir for 30-45 minutes.

6.   Filter the mixture and wash the filter cake with saline, appropriate buffers (pH 8.0, pH 2.4, etc., depending on the purpose), and finally with saline.

7.   Store the polymer in the form of wet filter cake in a freezer.

8.   For use disperse the polymer by using a loosely fitted (mismatched) tissue grinder (Potter-Elvehjem).

REFERENCES

1.   Avrameas, S. and Ternynck, T. Biologically active water-insoluble protein polymers. Their use for isolation of antigens and antibodies. *J. Biol. Chem.* *242*, 1651 (1967).

2.   ——————————. The cross-linking of proteins with glutaraldehyde and its use for the preparation of immunoadsorbents. *Immunochem. 6*, 53 (1969).

3.   Axen, R., Porath, J., and Ernback, S. Chemical coupling of peptides and proteins to polysaccharides by means of cyanogen halides. *Nature 214*, 1302 (1967).

4.   Campbell, D. H. and Weliky, N. Immunoadsorbents: Preparation and use cellulose derivatives. In C. A. Williams and M. W. Chase, Eds., *Methods in Immunology and Immunochemistry*, vol. 1, (Academic: New York 1967), p. 365.

5.   Carpenter, R. R. and Reisberg, M. A. Carbodiimide-induced bentonite-antigen complexes: Readily prepared immunoadsorbents. *J. Immunol. 100*, 873 (1968).

6.   Carrel, S. and Barrandun, S. Protein-containing polyacrylamide gels: Their use as immunoadsorbents of high capacity. *Immunochem. 8*, 39 (1971).

7.   Catt, K. J. and Tregear, G. W. Solid-phase radioimmunoassay in antibody coated tubes. *Science 158*, 1570 (1967).

8.   Centeno, E. R. and Sehon, A. H. High capacity immunoadsorbents prepared with ethylene-maleic anhydride copolymers. *Federation Proc. 25*, 729 (Abst.) (1966).

9.   Chidlow, J. W., Stephen, J., and Smith, H. Further studies on the specific and quantitative aspects of antigen adsorption by disulphide-linked antibody immunosorbents. *Immunochem. 7*, 505 (1970).

10.   Joniau, M., Onkelinx, E., and Lontie, R. Glutaraldehyde polymerized proteins as immunoadsorbents. *Arch. Int. Physiol. Biochem. 76*, 182 (1968).

11.   Kabat, E. A. and Mayer, M. M. *Experimental Immunochemistry*, 2nd ed. (Thomas: Springfield, Ill. 1961). p. 781.

12.   Levine, B. B. and Levytska, V. Hapten-specific immunoadsorbents prepared from hide powder (Collagen). *J. Immunol. 102*, 647 (1969).

13.   Onoue, K., Yagi, Y., and Pressman, D. Immunoadsorbents with high capacity. *Immunochem. 2*, 181 (1965).

14.   Robbins, J. B., Haimovich, J., and Sela, M. Purification of antibodies with immunoadsorbents prepared using bromacetylcellulose. *Immunochem. 4*, 11 (1967).

15.   Truffa-Bachi, P. and Wofsy, L. Specific separation of cells on affinity columns. *Proc. Natl. Acad. Sci. U. S. 66*, 685 (1970).

16.   Wide, J. and Porath, J. Radioimmunoassay of proteins with the use of Sephadex-coupled antibodies. *Biochim. Biophys. Acta 130*, 257 (1966).

QUANTITATIVE PROTEIN DETERMINATIONS

The protein content of a solution is usually measured in one of three ways: absorption of ultraviolet light; reactivity with color reagent (such as biuret reagent); and refractometry.

Ultraviolet Absorption

Protein containing solutions will absorb ultraviolet light in proportion to the amount of tyrosine, tryptophan, and/or phenylalanine present in the protein, and absorption is maximal at a wavelength of 280 nm.

The relationship between absorption and concentration is most usually expressed in the combined Beer-Lambert equation:

(1) $A = abc$

where

A = absorptivity (optical density = OD)
a = extinction coefficient (E)
b = optical path length
c = concentration

In effect this equation says that optical density varies linearly with concentration, all other factors being constant. It should be remembered that optical density is a logarithmic function of the light transmitted; the terms absorption (A) and transmission (T) are related thus: $A = -\log T$. They should not be confused.

Optical density (OD) is measured with a spectrophotometer, and concentration in percent (grams per 100 ml) is calculated from

(2) $C = OD/E$

This is simply equation (1) expressed in more familiar terms; b has been dropped from equation (1), since the optical path length of a standard cuvette is 1.00 cm.

It is not surprising that different proteins will absorb light in amounts differing with their content of tyrosine, tryptophan, and/or phenylalanine. The following list of extinction coefficients of some representative proteins illustrates that the content of these amino acids is by no means constant:

Protein	$E \, \dfrac{1 \, cm, \, 1\%}{280 \, nm}$
Bovine serum albumin	6.6
Human IgG	14.3
Human IgM	11.9
Human thyroglobulin	10.4

The chief drawback of this method is that it cannot be applied to mixtures whose makeup is unknown, since one does not know what extinction coefficient to use.

Coloring Method (Biuret)

Another method of estimating protein concentration involves the development of a colored compound that can be read at a given wavelength in a spectrophotometer when the protein is reacted with a specific reagent. The biuret reaction falls in this category and depends on the development of an intense purple color when Cu^{++} is added to an alkaline solution of protein. This reaction is specific for proteins and will not be given by free amino acids, small peptides, or nucleic acids. Since this reaction depends on structures in which there are several acid amides in close proximity (as provided by the peptide bond in proteins) and not on amino acid content, it can be applied to unknowns more readily than ultraviolet absorption, although it is not quite as sensitive.

Once E has been determined, C may be calculated as above, from spectrophotometer readings. E is essentially constant for most serum and soluble tissue proteins. (The Folin-Ciocalteu, or the Lowry Coloring Method will not be discussed here, as it has the drawback of depending on the aromatic amino acid content of the proteins, without the simplicity and reproducibility that are the redeeming factors of the ultraviolet absorption method.

Refractometry

The degree to which a beam of light is bent (refracted) when passing through a solution depends on the nature and extent of those substances present in the solution. Protein-containing solutions will refract light to the same degree, whether the protein in solution is BSA, IgG, or some other protein, provided the concentrations are the same. As concentration increases, the amount by which the light is refracted increases in a linear fashion (e.g., a 2% solution of BSA will refract light twice as much as a 1% solution of BSA). In general, this refractive index increment (Δn) is 0.00185, or

(3) $\Delta n = 0.00185$, for 1% increase in protein concentration.

Δn may be obtained from refractometer readings and converted to concentration by means of the 0.00185 factor.

As with the biuret reagent, separate factors are not needed for different proteins. An additional advantage of this method is that very small samples are required. But the method is limited to the differentiation of fairly high protein concentrations (more than 0.2%).

REFERENCE

1.   Schultze, H. E. and Heremans, J. F. *Molecular Biology of Human Proteins*, vol. I (Elsevier: New York, 1966), p. 100.

REAGENTS

ACETIC ACID 1M

(for amido black and Ponceau red stains)

Glacial acetic acid (17.4M)	57.7 ml
Distilled water to	1000 ml

AGAROSE, 1%, in BARBITAL BUFFER, pH 8.2

(for electroimmunodiffusion, crossed
electrophoresis, counterimmunoelectrophoresis)

1. Dissolve 3 g agarose in 150 ml distilled water. This can be done on a hot plate in a 500 ml Erlenmeyer flask, using a stirring bar. Increase the heat gradually until the solution is clear but do not allow the solution to boil. Add 150 ml barbital buffer (hot). Stir until the mixture is clear. Pour into tubes (16 ml each). Store at 4°C.
2. Melt a tube of 1% agarose in barbital buffer, pH 8.2. Place the tube in a beaker of water and heat over a low flame until the agarose is completely "sol." Avoid continued heating of the agarose to prevent hydrolysis and caramelization. Heating in a waterbath will reduce this risk.

AMIDO BLACK STAIN

(protein stain, for immunodiffusion, immunoelectrophoresis, etc.)

Amido black	1	g
1M acetic acid (p. 195)	500	ml
0.1M sodium acetate (p. 206)	500	ml

Dissolve dye in acetic acid, half volume at a time. Then add sodium acetate.

BARBITAL BUFFER, pH 8.2, ionic strength 0.05

(for immunoelectrophoresis, electroimmunodiffusion, crossed electrophoresis, counterimmunoelectrophoresis)

Sodium barbital	47.6	g
Distilled water	3	l
Mix and add:		
1.17N hydrochloric acid (HCl)	55.0	ml

Adjust pH to 8.2 with hydrochloric acid and make up to 4265 ml with distilled water (1.17N HCl = 193 ml concentrated HCl + 1807 ml distilled water).

BARBITAL BUFFER, $\Gamma/2$ = 0.05, pH 8.60

(for starch block electrophoresis)

Barbital	260	g
10N sodium hydroxide (NaOH)	122	ml
Distilled water	24	l

BENZIDINE SOLUTION

(for staining agar plates in hemolytic plaque technique)

Benzidine dihydrochloride	0.2 g
Distilled water	90.0 ml

Glacial acetic acid   10.0 ml
30% hydrogen peroxide   0.5 ml

The solution is stored at 4-6°C.

BIS-DIAZOTIZED BENZIDINE (BDB) SOLUTION

(for BDB hemagglutination)

1. Add 0.23 g of benzidine to 45 ml of 0.2N hydrochloric acid.
2. Add to this solution 0.175 g of sodium nitrate ($NaNO_2$) in 5 ml of distilled water at 4°C. Stir intermittently for half an hour.
3. Check this mixture with potassium iodide-starch indicator paper. The solution is good only if the paper turns deep blue.
4. Divide the solution into small aliquots of 0.5 ml (or less) amounts. A dry-ice-and-acetone bath is used to quick-freeze the solution, as it deteriorates quickly at room temperature. Keep in a freezer until ready for use. It is advisable to perform all the operations in a cold room.

BORATE BUFFER STOCK SOLUTION, pH 8.0

(for radioimmunoelectrophoresis, to wash slides)

Boric acid   12.37 g
Sodium hydroxide (pellets)   0.50 g
Sodium chloride   8.00 g
Distilled water to   1000   ml

Add distilled water just before use.

BOVINE SERUM ALBUMIN SOLUTION

(for complement fixation)

1. Prepare a 0.1 mg/ml stock solution of bovine serum albumin (BSA), crystalline (Nutritional Biochemical) in distilled water.
2. Prepare a 1:1000 dilution of stock BSA solution in phosphate-buffered saline, pH 7.2, before use.

BUFFERED GLYCEROL

(for immunofluorescence)

1. Prepare phosphate buffer, pH 8.0:
$0.1M Na_2 HPO_4$	94.5 ml
$0.1M NaH_2 PO_4$	5.5 ml
2. Combine and mix thoroughly nine volumes glycerol and one volume phosphate buffer, pH 8.0.

DESTAINING SOLUTION

(for Ponceau red and amido black staining)

Acetic acid	3.0 ml
Glycerol	10.0 ml
Distilled water	87.0 ml

DEXTRAN-COATED CHARCOAL (DCC) STOCK SUSPENSION

(for radioimmunoassays)

Suspend by magnetic stirring 10 g Norit A (neutral) charcoal in 100 ml 0.25% dextran in phosphate-buffered saline. Refrigerate. Stir magnetically in the cold before sampling and maintain under stirring during sampling.

ESTERASE STAINING

1. Indoxyl acetate solution
   A. Dissolve 5 mg indoxyl acetate in 0.5 ml acetone.
   B. Add 22 ml barbital buffer, pH 8.6 (p. 196).
   C. Add 2.5 ml of 10^{-3} M cupric acetate.
   D. Pour onto plate immediately.
2. β-naphthyl acetate-diazonium salt solution
   A. Dissolve 5 mg β-naphthyl acetate in 0.15 ml acetone. Add 13 ml of tris-HCl buffer, pH 7.4.
   B. Dissolve separately 10 mg diazo blue B in 12 ml of tris-HCl buffer, pH 7.4.

C.   Mix the two solutions and filter through paper before pouring onto the plate.

GELATIN VERONAL BUFFER (GVB=) 5X

Veronal-buffered saline (VB=)	100.0 ml
Gelatin (2%)	25.0 ml
Distilled water to	1000 ml

To prepare 2% gelatin, dissolve 10.0 g of gelatin in 500.0 ml commercially distilled water. Heat must be applied to dissolve the gelatin. This solution need not be prepared fresh. It can be stored cold and liquefied before use in a $37°C$ waterbath.

GVB= 5X has a shelf-life of one week when kept in the cold. Check the pH before use; if there is considerable pH change, make up fresh buffer.

GELATIN VERONAL BUFFER WITH Mg^{++} AND Ca^{++} (GVB^{++}) 2X

Veronal-buffered saline (VB=) 5X	200.0 ml
0.03M calcium chloride ($CaCl_2$)	10.0 ml*
0.10M magnesium chloride ($MgCl_2$)	10.0 ml*
2% gelatin	50.0 ml
Distilled water to	1000 ml

*Use a 10-ml volumetric pipette.

Add together and dilute in a volumetric flask. The pH should be 7.5.

To prepare 0.03M $CaCl_2$, dissolve 3.330 g $CaCl_2$ in 1000 ml of distilled water (commercial source).

To prepare 0.10M $MgCl_2$, dissolve 20.33 g of the hexahydrate $MgCl_2 \cdot 6H_2O$ in 1000 ml of commercially distilled water.

The two solutions (0.03M $CaCl_2$ and 0.10M $MgCl_2$) need not be prepared fresh: they can be stored in the cold.

GVB^{++} 2X has a shelf life of one week when kept in the cold. Check the pH before use: if there is considerable pH change, make up fresh buffer.

GLUCOSE-GELATIN VERONAL BUFFER with Mg^{++} and Ca^{++} (Gl-GVB^{++})

Mix equal volumes of the GVB^{++} (gelatin veronal buffer with Mg^{++} and Ca^{++}) and

5% glucose (Abbott 5% dextrose in H_2O or Baxter 5% dextrose in H_2O). The pH should be 7.5. This buffer, when kept cold, may be used for two days.

IONAGAR 0.5% IN 0.05M SODIUM CHLORIDE (NaCl) and 1.0% GLYCEROL

(for immunorheophoresis)

Ionagar no. 2 (Oxoid)	0.5 g
Glycerol	1.0 ml
NaCl, 0.05M to	100.0 ml

The glycerol is needed to keep the gel from drying out. The salt concentration of 0.05M is chosen so that a slight local increase in ionic strength close to the place of strongest evaporation will not create any disturbing effects. In practice the average increase in salt concentration in that place was no more than 15%, while the highest increase encountered remained under 25%. The much higher increase in protein concentration than in salt concentration between the wells is undoubtedly caused by the very low diffusivity of protein as compared to small ions.

ISOTONIC SODIUM EDTA SOLUTION, pH 7.4

1. Prepare 0.12M solution of disodium EDTA. Dissolve 44.66 g of dihydrated disodium EDTA (ethylenediaminetetracetic acid or ethylenedinitrilotetracetic acid) in 1000 ml of distilled water (commercial source). The pH should be 4.5.
2. Add 0.3N NaOH until the pH is 7.4. To prepare 0.3N NaOH, dilute 188 ml of Harleco 0.4 NaOH to 250 ml with commercially distilled water.

Note: To bring 500 ml of 0.12M EDTA to pH 7.4 requires approximately 190-200 ml of 0.3N NaOH.

3. Determine the final molarity of the sodium EDTA, pH 7.4, as follows:
    A.   Determination of dilution factor x:

$$x = \frac{\text{Starting volume of 0.12M EDTA } (Na_2), \text{ pH 4.5}}{\text{Final volume of EDTA } (Na_2), \text{ pH 7.4}}$$

B.   Determination of final molarity via the factor x:
(1)   Multiply dilution factor x by the original molarity of 0.12.
(2)   The final molarity (factor x) (0.12M) should be about 0.088M.

This solution need not be prepared fresh: it can be stored cold.

KARNOVSKY SOLUTION

(for peroxidase staining)

1.   Dissolve 75 mg of 3-3'diaminobenzidine in 100 ml tris-HCl, 0.05M, pH 7.6, stirring on a magnetic stirrer at room temperature in the dark for three hours.
2.   After three hours filter through Whatman no. 1 and store at 4°C. Make up fresh each time.
3.   Immediately before use add 1 ml of 0.3% H_2O_2 to 100 ml of diaminobenzidine solution (final concentration 0.003% H_2O).

LEUKOCYTES

(for leukocyte migration inhibition)

Materials

1.   Heparinized syringe, 30 ml, and 20 gauge needle
2.   Hanks Balanced Saline Solution (HBSS)
3.   Incubator, 37°C

Method

1.   Heparinized blood obtained by venipuncture is allowed to settle for 1 hour at 37°C.
2.   The buffy coat is removed, washed 4 times in HBSS and a 10% suspension is packed in capillary tubes.

LYMPHOCYTES

(for microdroplet lymphotoxicity test)

Materials

1. Patient's blood
2. Glass beads: 5 mm
3. Polyvinylpyrrolidone, 4% in PBS (PVP) (Type NP-K30, General Aniline and Film Corporation)
4. Cotton-tipped applicators
5. Anti-A, B blood grouping serum (Ortho Diagnostics)
6. Anti-H: made from Ulex Europaeus seeds (F. W. Schumacher Co., Sandwich, Mass.)
7. Fisher centrifuge tube
8. Fisher centrifuge Model 59
9. Plastic drinking straw: 6 x 100 mm
10. Nylon tricot
11. Glass beads: 0.2 mm diameter
12. Gum arabic powder
13. Rubber stoppers to fit 6 mm straw
14. Hanks' balanced saline solution (HBSS)
15. Hemocytometer

Method

1. Collect 15 ml of venous blood into a 125 ml Erlenmeyer flask containing 6 to 8 glass beads (5 mm diameter). Shake the flask gently in a circular motion until a clot forms around the glass beads. This will occur within 5 to 10 minutes.
2. Transfer the defibrinated blood to a 16 x 125 mm tube and add 1 ml of 4% PVP for each 4 ml of blood. Remove air bubbles and clean the inner glass surface with cotton swabs. Incubate the tube at a 45° angle in a 37°C waterbath for 15 minutes.
3. Remove the erythrocyte-poor, white blood cell-rich supernatant obtained from step 2, place it into a Kahn tube and centrifuge at 2500 rpm for 5 minutes in a clinical centrifuge.
4. Remove and save the clear supernatant. Resuspend the cell button in 3 to 5 drops of anti-A, B serum or anti-H reagent. Shake the tube gently until the contaminating red cells are strongly agglutinated. After addition of about 0.5 ml of the supernatant, transfer the suspension to a Fisher tube and spin

in the Fisher Microfuge for 1 to 2 seconds to sediment the agglutinates.

5.   Place the supernatant in a 10 cm column made from a plastic drinking straw which has been plugged at one end with nylon mesh and filled to ¾ volume with 0.2 mm glass beads pre-coated with 1% gum arabic. Stopper the column (watertight) and incubate for 5 minutes in a 37°C waterbath.

6.   The granulocytes adhere to the glass beads and purified lymphocytes are obtained by passing about 1 ml of HBSS through a column. Collect the lymphocyte suspension in a Fisher tube. Spin the tube at 500 g for 5 minutes in the Fisher Microfuge. Remove and discard the supernatant.

7.   Resuspend the cell button in about 0.5 ml of HBSS. Count the cells in a hemocytometer and adjust their concentration to 5,000 cells/μl.

(for macrophage migration inhibition)

Materials

1.   Sterile cotton fiber columns (e.g., Pasteur pipettes or glass syringes filled with cotton)
2.   50 ml heparinized syringe
3.   Incubator, 37°C
4.   Hanks' balanced saline solution (HBSS)

Method

1.   Draw 50 ml of blood by venipuncture into heparinized syringe and allow to sediment in the syringe in the upright position at 37°C.
2.   Remove the buffy coat containing the plasma and leukocytes and incubate in cotton fiber columns for 10 minutes at 37°C to remove monocytes and leukocytes. The cells which come through the columns are 90% lymphocytes.
3.   Wash lymphocytes in HBSS.

MACROPHAGES

(for macrophage migration inhibition)

Materials

1.   Young adult guinea pig (approximately 500-800 g)
2.   Sterile light mineral oil (Bayol-F)

3. Hanks' balanced saline solution (HBSS)
4. Culture medium, TC-199, with 15% normal guinea pug serum (heat-inactivated)
5. Separatory funnel, 250 ml
6. Cannulated trocar and plastic tubing
7. Syringes, 50 ml, and needles, 20 guage
8. Pipettes, 10 ml
9. Conical centrifuge bottle, 250 ml
10. Graduated centrifuge tubes, 10 ml
11. Refrigerated centrifuge

Method

1. Inject 30 ml sterile mineral oil into the abdominal cavity of the guinea pig. This induces a peritoneal exudate consisting of about 75% macrophages and 25% leukocytes.
2. Three to five days later sacrifice the animal by bleeding from the heart under ether anesthesia.
3. Inject 150 ml sterile HBSS into the abdominal cavity and knead the abdomen gently.
4. Drain the exudate into a separatory funnel by means of a cannulated trocar and plastic tubing.
5. Separate the HBSS and suspend cells from the oil.
6. Using a conical centrifuge bottle, centrifuge at 250 g for 10 minutes at 4°C to sediment the cells.
7. Resuspend the cell pellet in 10 ml of HBSS and wash twice.
8. Prepare a 10% suspension by volume in culture medium.

PHOSPHATE BUFFER, pH 8.0

(for radial immunodiffusion)

0.03M potassium phosphate
0.10M sodium chloride

PHOSPHATE BUFFER, pH 7.3, 0.15M

(for BDB cell hemagglutination and penicillin hemagglutination tests)

KH_2PO_4	20.41 g/l
Na_2HPO_4	21.30 g/l

To 100 ml of Na_2HPO_4, add 28 ml of KH_2PO_4 and adjust to pH 7.3.

PHOSPHATE-BUFFERED SALINE, pH 7.2

(for crossed electrophoresis)

Na_2HPO_4	1.48 g*
KH_2PO_4	0.43 g
NaCl	6.80 g

*Heat to dissolve.

Bring up to 1 liter with distilled water.

PHOSPHATE-BUFFERED SALINE, pH 7.4

(for digoxin radioimmunoassay)

K_2HPO_4	1.392 g
$NaH_2PO_4 \cdot H_2O$	0.276 g
NaCl	8.770 g

Dissolve in 900 ml distilled water. Adjust pH to 7.4 with 0.01N KOH and adjust final volume to 1000 ml.

PHOSPHATE-BUFFERED SALINE SOLUTION, pH 7.2, 0.15M

(tanned cell hemagglutination and BDB hemagglutination)

NaCl	36.0 g
Na_2HPO_4 (anhydrous)	7.4 g
KH_2PO_4 (anhydrous)	2.15 g

Make up to 5 liters in distilled water.

PONCEAU RED STAIN

   (protein stain, for immunodiffusion, immunoelectrophoresis, etc.)

Ponceau S   0.5 g
1M acetic acid (p. 195)   250.0 ml
0.1M sodium acetate (p. 206)   250.0 ml

Dissolve dye in acetic acid, half volume at a time. Then add sodium acetate.

SODIUM ACETATE 0.1M ($\cdot 3H_2O$)

   (for amido black and Ponceau red stains)

Sodium acetate hydrated ($\cdot 3H_2O$)   3.4 g
Distilled water to   250.0 ml
Or:
Sodium acetate (nonhydrated)   2.05 g
Distilled water to   250.0 ml

SODIUM BARBITAL BUFFER, pH 8.4

   (penicillin hemagglutination)

1.   Dissolve 2.06 g sodium barbital (sodium diethylbarbiturate) in 100 ml
     distilled water.
2.   Add 0.3 g NaCl to 82.3 ml sodium barbital solution.
3.   Adjust pH to 8.4 using 0.1N HCl (approximately 17.7 ml).

SODIUM ETHYLENEDIAMINETETRACETIC ACID-GELATIN VERONAL
BUFFER (EDTA-GVB=) with no calcium or magnesium ions, pH 7.4, 0.04M

   (for hemolytic C_4 assay)

1.   Prepare a 0.12M solution of disodium EDTA, pH 4.5 (44.66 g dihydrated
     disodium EDTA and distilled water up to 1000 ml).
2.   Add 0.3N NaOH to pH 7.4.

3.   Determine the final molarity of the disodium EDTA, pH 7.4 as follows:

$$M = \frac{\text{Starting volume of 0.12M disodium EDTA, pH 4.5}}{\text{Final volume of disodium EDTA, pH 7.4}} \; x \; \frac{\text{the original}}{\text{molarity (0.12M)}}$$

The final molarity should be approximately 0.088M.

4.   To make the disodium EDTA-GVB=, 0.040M, dilute the disodium EDTA solution, pH 7.4, molarity 0.088M, with GVB=. Calculate the volume of disodium EDTA to be diluted to 200 ml with GVB= as follows:

$$\frac{\text{volume of disodium EDTA}}{\text{to be diluted}} = \frac{(200) \quad (0.040)}{\text{final molarity of sodium EDTA, pH 7.4}}$$

This buffer has a shelf life of two days when kept refrigerated.

SPECIAL AGAR, 1%, in PBS

Ionagar no. 2 (Oxoid) or Noble Agar
(Difco) or Agarose (Bausch and Lomb)   1   g
Phosphate-buffered saline solution,
pH 7.2   100   ml

1.   Weigh out agar and place it in a 250-ml, wide-mouth Erlenmeyer flask.
2.   Add 90 ml saline solution and 10 ml thimerosal solution as a preservative (p. 209).
3.   Dissolve agar by heating in boiling-water bath or, preferably, in an auto-clave at 115°C.

SPECIAL AGAR, 3%, in PBS

Ionagar no. 2 (Oxoid) or Noble Agar
(Difco) or Agarose (Bausch and Lomb)   3   g
Phosphate-buffered saline solution,
pH 7.2   100   ml

1.   Weigh out agar and place it in a 250-ml wide-mouth Erlenmeyer flask.
2.   Add 90 ml saline solution and 10 ml thimerosal solution as a preservative (p. 209).

3.   Dissolve agar by heating in boiling-water bath or, preferably, in an auto-clave at 115°C.

SPECIAL AGAR, 1%, in Barbital Buffer

Ionagar no. 2 (Oxoid) or Noble Agar
(Difco) or Agarose (Bausch and Lomb)   1   g
Barbital acetate buffer $\Gamma/2 = 0.05$,
pH 8.2 (p. 196)   100   ml

TANNIC ACID SOLUTION

      (for tanned cell hemagglutination)

Tannic acid (Mallenckrodt fluffy)   0.1 g

Dissolve in 20 ml distilled water.
      This stock solution may be kept for 1 week.
      For use in test, dilute 1:125 in PBS.

TAP BUFFER (Electro-Nucleonics Laboratories, Inc.)

      (HA antibody hemagglutination)

1. $0.2M\ NaH_2PO_4$ 115.0 ml
      $0.2M\ Na_2HPO_4$ 385.0 ml
      NaCl   17.0 g
      Polyvinylpyrrolidone (PVP)   50.0 mg
      Tween 80   0.1 ml
      Sodium azidide   2.0 g

      Add the above in a 2000-ml volumetric flask and dilute with distilled water.
2.   5.0 ml of a 5% solution of bovine serum albumin in saline (aliquots can be stored at −20°C) is diluted into 45.0 ml of the phosphate buffer (TAP buffer) for use. This combined buffer can be stored at 2-8°C for several weeks.

THIMEROSAL SOLUTION

Dilute merthiolate (thimerosal, Eli Lilly Co.) 1:1000 in saline.

THYROID EXTRACT

(for tanned cell hemagglutination)

1. Infuse an equal amount (weight/volume) of minced human thyroid tissue with PBS overnight.
2. Centrifuge at 64,000 g for 45 minutes and pass through millipore HA filter. Sterile thyroid extract can be stored in the refrigerator for several weeks.

TRIETHANOLAMINE-BUFFERED SALINE (TEAE), pH 7.3-7.4

(complement-fixation test)

1. 10 X stock solution (1 l):

Triethanolamine	28.0 ml
HCl 1N	180.0 ml
NaCl	75.0 g
$MgCl_2 \cdot 6H_2O$ (MW 203.31)	1.0 g
$CaCl_2 \cdot 2H_2O$ (MW 147.02)	0.2 g

2. For working solution, isotonic, $\Gamma/2 = 0.15$, dilute stock solution with nine volumes of distilled water to provide 5×10^4 Mg^{++} and 1.5×10^4 M Ca^{++}.

VERONAL-BUFFERED SALINE (VB=) 5X

NaCl	83.0 g
Sodium barbital ($NaC_8H_{11}N_2O_3$)	10.19 g

Dissolve in about 1500 ml of distilled water (from a commercial source). Add 34.6 ml of 1.0N HCl. The pH should be 7.3. Dilute to 2000 ml in a 2-l volumetric flask.

Index